THE TIBETAN YOGAS OF DREAM AND SLEEP

Tenzin Wangyal Rinpoche

Edited by
Mark Dahlby

Snow Lion Publications
Ithaca, New York

Snow Lion Publications
P.O. Box 6483
Ithaca, New York 14851 USA
607-273-8519

Printed in Canada on acid-free recycled paper.

ISBN 1-55939-101-4

Libary of Congress Cataloging-in-Publication Data

Wangyal, Tenzin.
    Tibetan yogas of dream and sleep / Tenzin Wangyal Rinpoche ; edited
by Mark Dahlby.
        p.   cm.
    Includes bibliographical references.
    ISBN 1-55939-101-4 (alk. paper)
    1. Yoga (Bonpo) 2. Dreams--Religious aspects--Bonpo (Sect) 3. Sleep--
Religious aspects--Bonpo (Sect) I. Dahlby, mark. II. Title.
    BQ7982.2.W36 1998
    294.3'4446--dc21   98-23380
                                                                               CIP

THE TIBETAN YOGAS
OF DREAM AND SLEEP

Table of Contents

Acknowledgments

I want to thank the people who have been instrumental in bringing this book to publication. First of all, and most importantly, Mark Dahlby, my student and close friend, with whom I greatly enjoyed working. We spent many hours discussing different issues in cafes around Berkeley. Without him, this book would not have been possible.

Also: Steven D. Goodman, a colleague and friend, improved the manuscript through numerous good suggestions; Sue Ellis Dyer and Chris Baker made editing suggestions on an early version of the book; Sue Davis and Laura Shekerjian helped by reading the text and offering feedback; and Christine Cox of Snow Lion Publications brought her great skill as an experienced editor to the text and made it a much better book.

The photographs of the meditation and dream yoga positions, on pages 85 and 109 respectively, were taken by Antonio Riestra and modeled by Luz Vergara. The illustrations of the chakras on pages 105 and 107 were created by Monica R. Ortega. I also want to thank all those I have not named but who have helped in many different ways.

This book is dedicated to Namkhai Norbu Rinpoche,
who has been a great inspiration in my life,
both in how I teach others and in my own practice.

Preface

A well-known saying in Tibetan states, "One should explain the lineage and the history in order to cut doubt about the authenticity of the teaching and the transmission." Therefore, I begin this book with a short story of my life.

I was born shortly after my parents fled the Chinese oppression in Tibet. Conditions were difficult and my parents placed me in a Christian boarding school, where they hoped I would be cared for. My father was a Buddhist *lama**, my mother a practitioner of Bön*. Some time after, my father died. Eventually my mother remarried a man who was a Bön lama. Both he and my mother desired that I live within my culture, and when I was ten years old I was taken to the main Bön monastery in Dolanji, India, and ordained as a monk.

After living in the monastery for some time, I was recognized by Lopon (Head Teacher) Sangye Tenzin Rinpoche as the reincarnation of Khyungtul Rinpoche, a famous scholar, teacher, author, and meditation master. He was well known as a master astrologer, and in western Tibet and northern India was famous as a tamer of wild spirits. He was widely sought after as a healer with magical abilities. One of his sponsors was a local king of Himachal in Northern India. This king and his wife, unable to bear children, asked Khyungtul Rinpoche to heal them, which he did. The son that they bore and raised is the present day Chief Minister of Himachal Pradesh, Virbhardur.

When I was thirteen, my kind root master, Lopon Sangye Tenzin, a man of great knowledge and realization, prepared to teach one of the most important and esoteric teachings in the Bön religion: the Great Perfection (Dzogchen*) lineage of the Oral Transmission of Zhang Zhung (Zhang Zhung Nyan Gyud*). Even though I was still young, my step-father visited Lopon Rinpoche and asked that I be admitted to the teachings, which would take place every day for three years. Lopon kindly agreed, but asked that I, along with the other prospective students, bring him a dream from the night before the teachings were to begin, so that he might determine our readiness.

Some of the students remembered no dream, which was considered a sign of obstacles. Lopon had them begin appropriate purification practices and delayed the beginning of the teaching until each student did have a dream. Dreams of other students were taken as indications that they needed to do particular practices to ready themselves for the teachings—for example, doing practices that strengthened their connections to the Bön guardians*.

I dreamt about a bus circumambulating my teacher's house, although there is actually no road there. In the dream, the bus conductor was my friend and I stood beside him, handing out tickets to each person that boarded the bus. The tickets were pieces of paper that had the Tibetan syllable A written on them. That was in the second or third year of my education at Dolanji, when I was thirteen years old, and at the time I did not know that A was a symbol of major significance in Dzogchen teachings. My teacher never said anything about the dream, which was his way. He made little comment about what was good, but I was happy as long as I was allowed to come to the teachings.

It is common, in Tibetan spiritual traditions, for dreams of the students to be used by the teacher in this fashion to determine if it is appropriate for a student to receive a particular teaching. Though it would be some time before I began to study and practice dream yoga, this incident was the beginning of my interest in dreams. It strongly impressed on me how greatly dream is valued in Tibetan culture and in the Bön religion, and how information from the unconscious is often of greater value than the information the conscious mind can provide.

After the three-year teaching, which included numerous meditation retreats with my fellow practitioners as well as many retreats that I did alone, I entered the monastic Dialectic School. The program of study normally takes nine to thirteen years to complete and covers the traditional training. We were taught the common academic subjects, such as grammar, Sanskrit, poetry, astrology, and art, and also learned the uncommon subjects: epistemology, cosmology, sutra*, *tantra** and Dzogchen. During the monastic training, I was exposed to a number of teachings and transmissions on dream, the most important based on the texts of the Zhang Zhung Nyan Gyud, the Mother Tantra, and of Shardza Rinpoche.

I did well in the training and when I was nineteen I was asked to begin teaching others, which I did. Around the same time I wrote and published a summary of the biography of Lord Shenrab Miwoche*, the founder of the Bön religion. Later I became the president of the Dialectic School and held that position for four years, and was very involved in shaping and developing the school. In 1986, I received the *Geshe* degree, the highest degree awarded in Tibetan monastic education.

In 1989, at the invitation of Namkhai Norbu Rinpoche's Dzogchen Community in Italy, I traveled to the West. Although I had no plans to teach, I was invited to do so by members of the community. One day I was passing out small pieces of paper to be used in a meditation on concentration. Each piece of paper had the Tibetan syllable *A* written on it. Right then the dream from fifteen years before, in which I passed out the same paper to people getting on the bus, came back to me. It was as if it hit me on the head.

I remained in the West and in 1991 was awarded a Rockefeller Fellowship to do research at Rice University. In 1993, I published my first book in the West, *The Wonders of the Natural Mind*, in which I tried to present the Great Perfection (Dzogchen) teachings in a clear and simple way. In 1994 I was given a grant from The National Endowment for the Humanities to pursue research on the logical and philosophical aspects of the Bön tradition, in collaboration with Professor Anne Klein, Chair of Religious Studies, at Rice University.

So my scholarly side has continued to manifest, but practice is always more important, and during all this time I have been interested in dream and dream practice. My interest is not only theoretical. I have trusted the wisdom of my dreams, influenced from an early age by the dream experiences of my teachers and my mother and by the use of dreams in the Bön tradition, and I have been practicing dream yoga intensively during the last ten years. Every night when I get into bed, I feel freedom. The busyness of the day is over. Some nights the practice is successful and some nights it is not, and that is to be expected until the practice is very advanced. Nevertheless, I go to sleep nearly every night with the intention to accomplish dream practice. It is from my own experience with the practice, as well as from the three texts that I quote above, that the teachings in this book come.

The Tibetan Yogas of Dream and Sleep grew out of oral teachings I gave in California and New Mexico over several years. Much of the informality that was part of the teachings has been kept. Words marked with an asterisk upon their first appearance in the text can be found in the glossary at the back of the book.

Dream yoga is a primary support in developing my own practice and this has been true for many, many masters and yogis* of Tibet. For example, I have always been impressed with the story of Shardza Rinpoche, a great Tibetan master who, when he died in 1934, attained the body of light (*jalus**), a sign of full realization. During his life he had many accomplished students, wrote many important texts, and worked for the benefit of the country in which he lived. It's difficult to imagine how he could have been so productive in his external life, fulfilling the many responsibilities and long projects he undertook for the benefit of others, and still have been able to accomplish such attainment through spiritual practice. He could do this because he was not a writer for part of the day, a teacher for another part, and a practitioner for the few hours left. All of his life was practice, whether he was sitting in meditation, writing, teaching, or sleeping. He writes that dream practice was of central importance in his spiritual journey and integral to his attainment. This can also be true for us.

Introduction

We spend a third of our life sleeping. No matter what we do, however virtuous or non-virtuous our activities, whether we are murderers or saints, monks or libertines, every day ends the same. We shut our eyes and dissolve into darkness. We do so fearlessly, even as everything we know as "me" disappears. After a brief period, images arise and our sense of self arises with them. We exist again in the apparently limitless world of dream. Every night we participate in these most profound mysteries, moving from one dimension of experience to another, losing our sense of self and finding it again, and yet we take it all for granted. We wake in the morning and continue in "real" life, but in a sense we are still asleep and dreaming. The teachings tell us that we can continue in this deluded, dreamy state, day and night, or wake up to the truth.

When we engage in sleep and dream yogas we become part of a long lineage. Men and women have—for centuries—done these same practices, confronted the same doubts and obstacles that we do, and received the same benefits that we can. Many high lamas and accomplished yogis have made sleep and dream yogas primary practices, and through them have attained realization. Reflecting on this history and remembering the people who have dedicated their lives to the teachings—our spiritual ancestors who through these teachings pass to us the fruits of their practice—will generate faith in and gratitude for the tradition.

Some Tibetan masters might find it strange that I teach these practices to Westerners who have not done certain preliminary practices or who do not have certain understandings. The teachings were traditionally maintained as secret teachings, both as a sign of respect and as a protection against dilution through the misunderstanding of unprepared practitioners. They were never taught publicly nor given lightly, but were reserved for individuals who had prepared to receive them.

The practices are no less efficacious and valuable then they ever were, but conditions in the world have changed, and so I am trying something different. I hope that by teaching what is effective, openly and simply, the tradition will be better preserved and more people will be able to benefit from it. But it is important to respect the teachings, both to protect them and to further our own practice. Please try to receive the direct transmission of these teachings from an authentic teacher. It is good to read about these yogas but better to receive the oral transmission, which creates a stronger connection with the lineage. Also, it is easy to encounter obstacles on the path that are hard to overcome on our own but which an experienced teacher can identify and help to remove. This is an important point that should not be forgotten.

Our human lives are precious. We have intact bodies and minds, with complete potential. We may have met teachers and received teachings, and we have lives in which we enjoy the freedom to follow the spiritual path. We know that practice is essential to the spiritual journey as well as to our aspiration to help others. We also know life passes quickly and death is certain, yet in our busy lives we find it difficult to practice as much as we wish we could. Perhaps we meditate for an hour or two each day, but that leaves the other twenty-two hours in which to be distracted and tossed about on the waves of *samsara**. But there is always time for sleep; the third of our lives we spend sleeping can be used for practice.

A main theme of this book is that through practice we can cultivate greater awareness during every moment of life. If we do, freedom and flexibility continually increase and we are less governed by habitual preoccupations and distractions. We develop a stable and vivid presence that allows us to more skillfully choose positive responses to whatever arises, responses that best benefit others and our own spiritual journey. Eventually we develop a continuity of awareness that allows us to maintain full awareness during dream as well as in waking life. Then we are able to respond to dream phenomena in creative and positive ways and can accomplish various practices in the dream state. When we fully develop this capacity, we will find that we are living both waking and dreaming life with greater ease, comfort, clarity, and appreciation, and we will also be preparing ourselves to attain liberation in the intermediate state (*bardo**) after death.

The teachings provide us with many methods to improve the quality of ordinary life. That is good, for this life is important and worthwhile. But always the ultimate use of these yogas is to lead us to liberation. To that end, this book is best understood as a practice manual, a guide to the yogas of the Bön-Buddhist traditions of Tibet that use dreams to attain liberation from the dreaminess of ordinary life and use sleep to wake from ignorance. To use the book this way, you should make a connection with a qualified teacher. Then, to stabilize the mind, do the practices of calm abiding (*zhiné**) found in Part Three. When you feel ready, begin the preliminary practices and spend some time with them, integrating them into your life. Then begin the primary practices.

There is no hurry. We have wandered in the illusions of samsara for time without beginning. To simply read another book about spirituality and then forget it will change little in life. But if we follow these practices to their end, we will wake to our primordial nature, which is enlightenment itself.

If we cannot remain present during sleep, if we lose ourselves every night, what chance do we have to be aware when death comes? If we enter our dreams and interact with the mind's images as if they are real, we should not expect to be free in the state after death. Look to your experience in dreams to know how you will fare in death. Look to your experience of sleep to discover whether or not you are truly awake.

RECEIVING THE TEACHINGS

The best approach to receiving oral and written spiritual teachings is to "hear, conclude, and experience," that is, intellectually understand what is said, conclude what is meant, and apply it in practice. If learning is approached this way, the process of learning is continuous and unceasing, but if it stops at the level of the intellect, it can become a barrier to practice.

As to hearing or receiving the teachings, the good student is like a glue-covered wall: weeds thrown against it stick to it. A bad student is like a dry wall: what is tossed against it slides to the floor. When the teachings are received, they should not be lost or wasted. The student should retain the teachings in his or her mind, and work with them. Teachings not penetrated with understanding are like weeds thrown against the dry wall; they fall to the floor and are forgotten.

Coming to the conclusion of the meaning of teachings is like turning on a light in a dark room: what was hidden becomes clear. It is the experience of "a-ha!" when the pieces click into place and are understood. It's different from simple conceptual understanding in that it is something we know rather than something we have merely heard. For example, being told about yellow and red cushions in a room is like gaining an intellectual understanding of them, but if we go into the room when it is dark, we cannot tell which cushion is which. Concluding the meaning is like turning the light on: then we directly know the red and the yellow. The teaching is no longer something we can only repeat, it is part of us.

By "applying in practice," we mean turning what has been conceptually understood—what has been received, pondered, and made meaningful—into direct experience. This process is analogous to tasting salt. Salt can be talked about, its chemical nature understood, and so on, but the direct experience is had when it is tasted. That experience cannot be grasped intellectually and cannot be conveyed in words. If we try to explain it to someone who has never tasted salt, they will not be able to understand what it is that we have experienced. But when we talk of it to someone who already has had the experience, then we both know what is being referred to. It is the same with the teachings. This is how to study them: hear or read them, think about them, conclude the meaning, and find the meaning in direct experience.

In Tibet, new leather skins are put in the sun and rubbed with butter to make them softer. The practitioner is like the new skin, tough and hard with narrow views and conceptual rigidity. The teaching (*dharma**) is like the butter, rubbed in through practice, and the sun is like direct experience; when both are applied the practitioner becomes soft and pliable. But butter is also stored in leather bags. When butter is left in a bag for some years, the leather of the bag becomes hard as wood and no amount of new butter can soften it. Someone who spends many years studying the teachings, intellectualizing a great deal with little experience of practice, is like that hardened leather. The teachings can soften the hard skin of ignorance and conditioning, but when they are stored in the intellect and not rubbed into the practitioner with practice and warmed with direct experience, that person may become rigid and hard in his intellectual understanding. Then new teachings will not soften him, will not penetrate and change him. We must be careful not to store up the teachings as only conceptual understanding lest that conceptual understanding becomes a block to wisdom. The teachings are not ideas to be collected, but a path to be followed.

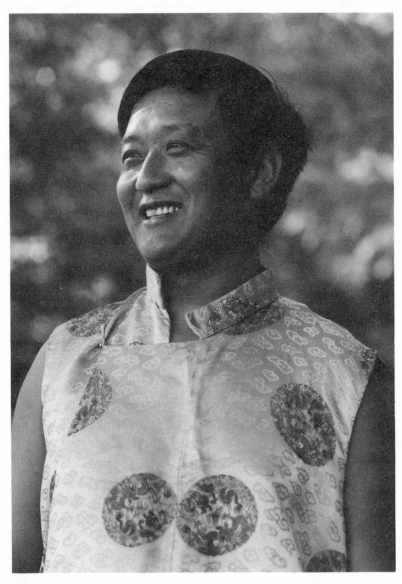

Tenzin Wangyal Rinpoche

PART ONE

The Nature of Dream

1 Dream and Reality

All of us dream whether we remember dreaming or not. We dream as infants and continue dreaming until we die. Every night we enter an unknown world. We may seem to be our ordinary selves or someone completely different. We meet people whom we know or don't know, who are living or dead. We fly, encounter non-human beings, have blissful experiences, laugh, weep, and are terrified, exalted, or transformed. Yet we generally pay these extraordinary experiences little attention. Many Westerners who approach the teachings do so with ideas about dream based in psychological theory; subsequently, when they become more interested in using dream in their spiritual life, they usually focus on the content and meaning of dreams. Rarely is the nature of dreaming itself investigated. When it is, the investigation leads to the mysterious processes that underlie the whole of our existence, not only our dreaming life.

The first step in dream practice is quite simple: one must recognize the great potential that dream holds for the spiritual journey. Normally the dream is thought to be "unreal," as opposed to "real" waking life. But there is nothing more real than dream. This statement only makes sense once it is understood that normal waking life is as unreal as dream, and in exactly the same way. Then it can be understood that dream yoga applies to all experience, to the dreams of the day as well as the dreams of the night.

2 How Experience Arises

IGNORANCE

All of our experience, including dream, arises from ignorance. This is a rather startling statement to make in the West, so first let us understand what is meant by ignorance (*ma-rigpa**). The Tibetan tradition distinguishes between two kinds of ignorance: innate ignorance and cultural ignorance. Innate ignorance is the basis of samsara, and the defining characteristic of ordinary beings. It is ignorance of our true nature and the true nature of the world, and it results in entanglement with the delusions of the dualistic mind.

Dualism reifies polarities and dichotomies. It divides the seamless unity of experience into this and that, right and wrong, you and me. Based on these conceptual divisions, we develop preferences that manifest as grasping and aversion, the habitual responses that make up most of what we identify as ourselves. We want this, not that; believe in this, not that; respect this and disdain that. We want pleasure, comfort, wealth, and fame, and try to escape from pain, poverty, shame, and discomfort. We want these things for ourselves and those we love, and do not care about others. We want an experience different from the one we are having, or we want to hold on to an experience and avoid the inevitable changes that will lead to its cessation.

There is a second kind of ignorance that is culturally conditioned. It comes about as desires and aversions become institutionalized in a culture and codified into value systems. For example, in India, Hindus believe that it is wrong to eat cows but proper to eat pigs. Moslems believe that it is appropriate to eat beef but they are prohibited from eating pork. Tibetans eat both. Who is right? The Hindu thinks the Hindus are right, the Moslem thinks the Moslems are right, and the Tibetan thinks the Tibetans are right. The differing beliefs arise from the biases and beliefs that are part of the culture—not from fundamental wisdom.

Another example can be found in the internal conflicts of philosophy. There are many philosophical systems that are defined by their disagreement with one another on fine points. Even though the systems themselves are developed with the intention to lead beings to wisdom, they produce ignorance in that their followers cling to a dualistic understanding of reality. This is unavoidable in any conceptual system because the conceptual mind itself is a manifestation of ignorance.

Cultural ignorance is developed and preserved in traditions. It pervades every custom, opinion, set of values, and body of knowledge. Both individuals and cultures accept these preferences as so fundamental that they are taken to be common sense or divine law. We grow up attaching ourselves to various beliefs, to a political party, a medical system, a religion, an opinion about how things should be. We pass through elementary school, high school, and maybe college, and in one sense every diploma is an award for developing a more sophisticated ignorance. Education reinforces the habit of seeing the world through a certain lens. We can become an expert in an erroneous view, become very precise in our understanding, and relate to other experts. This can be the case also in philosophy, in which one learns detailed intellectual systems and develops the mind into a sharp instrument of inquiry. But until innate ignorance is penetrated, one is merely developing an acquired bias, not fundamental wisdom.

We become attached to even the smallest things: a particular brand of soap or our hair being cut in a certain fashion. On a grand scale, we develop religions, political systems, philosophies, psychologies, and sciences. But no one is born with the belief that it is wrong to eat beef or pork or that one philosophical system is right and the other in error or that this religion is true and that religion is false. These must be learned. The allegiance to particular values is the result of cultural ignorance, but the propensity to accept limited views originates in the dualism that is the manifestation of innate ignorance.

This is not bad. It is just what is. Our attachments can lead to war but they also manifest as helpful technologies and different arts that are of great benefit to the world. As long as we are unenlightened we participate in dualism, and that is all right. In Tibetan there is a saying, "When in the body of a donkey, enjoy the taste of grass." In other words, we should appreciate and enjoy this life because it is meaningful and valuable in itself, and because it is the life we are living.

If we are not careful, the teachings can be used to support our ignorance. One can say that it is bad for someone to get an advanced degree, or wrong to have dietary restrictions, but this is not the point at all. Or one might say that ignorance is bad or normal life is only samsaric stupidity. But ignorance is simply an obscuration of consciousness. Being attached to it or repelled by it is just the same old game of dualism, played out in the realm of ignorance. We can see how pervasive it is. Even the teachings must work with dualism—by encouraging attachment to virtue, for example, and aversion to non-virtue—paradoxically using the dualism of ignorance to overcome ignorance. How subtle our understanding must become and how easily we can get lost! This is why practice is necessary, in order to have direct experience rather than just developing another conceptual system to elaborate and defend. When things are seen from a higher perspective they tend to level out. From the perspective of non-dual wisdom there is no important and unimportant.

ACTIONS AND RESULTS: KARMA AND KARMIC TRACES

The culture in which we live conditions us, but we carry the seeds of conditioning with us wherever we go. Everything that bothers us is actually in our mind. We blame our unhappiness on the environment, our situation, and believe that if we could change our circumstances we would be happy. But the situation in which we find ourselves is only the secondary cause of our suffering. The primary cause is innate ignorance and the resulting desire for things to be other than they are.

Perhaps we decide to escape the stresses of the city by moving to the ocean or the mountains. Or we may leave the isolation and difficulties of the country for the excitement of the city. The change can be nice because the secondary causes are altered and contentment may be found. But only for a short while. The root of our discontent moves with us to our new home, and from it grow new dissatisfactions. Soon we are once again caught up in the turmoil of hope and fear.

Or we may think that if we just had more money, or a better partner, or a better body or job or education, we would be happy. But we know this is not true. The rich are not free from suffering, a new partner will dissatisfy us in some way, the body will age, the new job will grow less interesting, and so on. When we think the solution to our unhappiness can be found in the external world, our desires can only be temporarily sated. Not understanding this, we are tossed this way and that by the winds of desire, ever restless and dissatisfied. We are governed by our karma and continually plant the seeds of future karmic harvest. Not only does this mode of action distract us from the spiritual path, but it also prevents us from finding satisfaction and happiness in our daily life.

As long as we identify with the grasping and aversion of the moving mind, we produce the negative emotions that are born in the gap between what is and what we want. Actions generated from these emotions, which include nearly all actions taken in our ordinary lives, leave karmic traces.

Karma* means action. Karmic traces* are the results of actions, which remain in the mental consciousness and influence our future. We can partially understand karmic traces if we think of them as what in the West are called tendencies in the unconscious. They are inclinations, patterns of internal and external behavior, ingrained reactions, habitual conceptualizations. They dictate our emotional reactions to situations and our intellectual understandings as well as our characteristic emotional habits and intellectual rigidities. They create and condition every response we normally have to every element of our experience.

This is an example of karmic traces on a gross level, though the same dynamic is at work in even the subtlest and most pervasive levels of experience: A man grows up in a home in which there is a lot of fighting. Then, perhaps thirty or forty years after leaving home, he is walking down a street and passes a house in which people are arguing with one another. That night he has a dream in which he is fighting with his wife or partner. When he wakes in the morning he feels aggrieved and withdrawn. This is noticed by his partner who reacts to the mood, which further irritates him.

This sequence of experiences shows us something about karmic traces. When the man was young, he reacted to the fighting in his home with fear, anger, and hurt. He felt aversion toward the fighting, a normal response, and this aversion left a trace in his mind. Decades later he passes a house and hears fighting; this is the secondary condition that stimulates the old karmic trace, which manifests in a dream that night.

In the dream, the man reacts to the dream-partner's provocation with feelings of anger and hurt. This response is governed by the karmic traces that were collected in his mental consciousness as a child and that have probably been reinforced many times since. When the dream-partner—who is wholly a projection of the man's mind—provokes him, his reaction is aversion, just as when he was a child. The aversion that he feels in the dream is the new action that creates a new seed. When he wakes he is stuck in the negative emotions that are the fruit of prior karmas; he feels estranged and withdrawn from his partner. To complicate matters further, the partner reacts from her karmically determined habitual tendencies, perhaps becoming short-tempered, withdrawn, apologetic, or subservient, and the man again reacts negatively, sowing yet another karmic seed.

Any reaction to any situation—external or internal, waking or dreaming—that is rooted in grasping or aversion, leaves a trace in the mind. As karma dictates reactions, the reactions sow further karmic seeds, which further dictate reactions, and so on. This is how karma leads to more of itself. It is the wheel of samsara, the ceaseless cycle of action and reaction.

Although this example focuses on karma on the psychological level, karma determines every dimension of existence. It shapes the emotional and mental phenomena in an individual's life as well as the perception and interpretation of existence, the functioning of the body, and the cause and effect dynamism of the external world. Every aspect of experience, however small or large, is governed by karma.

The karmic traces left in the mind are like seeds. And like seeds, they require certain conditions in order to manifest. Just as a seed needs the right combination of moisture and light and nutrients and temperature in order to sprout and grow, the karmic trace manifests when the right situation is encountered. The elements of the situation that support the manifestation of the karma are known as the secondary causes and conditions.

It is helpful to think of karma as the process of cause and effect, because this leads to the recognition that the choices made in responding to any situation, internal or external, have consequences. Once we really understand that each karmic trace is a seed for further karmically governed action, we can use that understanding to avoid creating negativity in our life, and instead create conditions that will influence our lives in a positive direction. Or, if we know how, we can allow the emotion to self-liberate as it arises, in which case no new karma is created.

NEGATIVE KARMA

If we react to a situation with negative emotion, the trace left in the mind will eventually ripen and influence a situation in life negatively. For example, if someone is angry with us and we in turn react with anger, we leave a trace that makes it more likely for anger to arise in us again, and furthermore it becomes more likely for us to encounter the secondary situations which allow our habitual anger to arise. This is easy to see if we have a great deal of anger in our lives or if we know someone who does. Angry people continually encounter situations that seem to justify their anger, while people with less anger do not. The external situations may be similar but the different karmic inclinations create different subjective worlds.

If an emotion is expressed impulsively it can generate strong results and reactions. Anger can lead to a fight or some other kind of destruction. People can be harmed physically or emotionally. This is not true just of anger; if fear is acted out it too can create great stress for the person who suffers it, can alienate that person from others, and so on. It is not too difficult to see how this leads to negative traces that influence the future negatively.

If we suppress emotion, there is still a negative trace. Suppression is a manifestation of aversion. It occurs through tightening something inside of ourselves, putting something behind a door and locking it, forcing part of our experience into the dark where it waits, seemingly hostile, until the appropriate secondary cause calls it out. This may manifest in many ways. For example, if we suppress our jealousy of others, it may eventually manifest in an emotional outburst, or it may be present in the harsh judgment of others of whom we are secretly jealous, even if we deny this jealousy to ourselves. Mental judgment is also an action, based on aversion, that creates negative karmic seeds.

POSTIVE KARMA

Instead of either of these negative responses—being driven in our behavior by the karmic tendency or suppressing it—we can take a moment to stop and communicate with ourselves and choose to produce the antidote to the negative emotion. If someone is angry with us and our own anger arises, the antidote is compassion. Inducing it may feel forced and inauthentic at first, but if we realize that the person irritating us is being pushed around by his own conditioning, and further realize that he is suffering a constriction of consciousness because he is trapped in his own negative karma, we feel some compassion and can start to let go of our negative reactions. As we do, we begin to shape our future positively.

This new response, which is still based on desire—in this case for virtue or peace or spiritual growth—produces a karmic trace that is positive; we have planted the seed of compassion. The next time we encounter anger we are a little more likely to respond with compassion, which is much more comfortable and spacious than the narrowness of self-protective anger. In this way, the practice of virtue cumulatively retrains our response to the world and we find ourselves, for instance, encountering less and less anger both internally and externally. If we continue in this practice, compassion will eventually arise spontaneously and without effort. Using the understanding of karma, we can retrain our minds to use all experience, even the most private and fleeting daydreams, to support our spiritual practice.

LIBERATING EMOTIONS

The best response to negative emotion is to allow it to self-liberate by remaining in non-dual awareness, free of grasping and aversion. If we can do this, the emotion passes through us like a bird flying through space; no trace of its passage remains. The emotion arises and then spontaneously dissolves into emptiness.

In this case, the karmic seed is manifesting—as emotion or thought or bodily sensation or an impulse toward particular behaviors—but because we do not respond with grasping or aversion, no seed of future karma is generated. Every time that envy, for example, is allowed to arise and dissolve in awareness without our becoming caught by it or trying to repress it, the strength of the karmic tendency toward envy weakens. There is no new action to reinforce it. Liberating emotion in this way cuts karma at its root. It is as if we burn the karmic seeds before they have an opportunity to grow into trouble in our life.

You may ask why it is better to liberate emotion rather than to generate positive karma. The answer is that all karmic traces act to constrain us, to restrict us to particular identities. The goal of the path is complete liberation from all conditioning. This does not mean that, once one is liberated, positive traits such as compassion are not present. They are. But when we are no longer driven by karmic tendencies we can see our situation clearly and respond spontaneously and appropriately, rather than being pushed in one direction or pulled in another. The relative compassion that arises from positive karmic tendencies is very good, but better is the absolute compassion that arises effortlessly and perfectly in the individual liberated from karmic conditioning. It is more spacious and inclusive, more effective, and free of the delusions of dualism.

Although allowing emotion to self-liberate is the best response, it is difficult to do before our practice is developed and stable. But however our practice is now, all of us can determine to stop for a moment when emotion arises, check in with ourselves, and choose to act as skillfully as possible. We can all learn to blunt the force of impulse, of karmic habits. We can use a conceptual process, reminding ourselves that the emotion we are experiencing is simply the fruition of previous karmic traces. Then we may be able to relax our identification with the emotion or point of view, and let go of our defensiveness. As the knot of emotion loosens, the identity relaxes and grows more spacious. We can choose a more positive response, planting seeds of positive karma. Again, it is important to do this without repressing emotion. We should relax as we generate compassion, not rigidly suppress the anger in our body while trying to think good thoughts.

The spiritual journey is not meant to benefit only the far future or our next life. As we practice training ourselves to react more positively to situations, we change our karmic traces and develop qualities that effect positive changes in the lives we are leading right now. As we see more clearly that every experience, however small and private, has a result, we can use this understanding to change our lives and our dreams.

OBSCURATIONS OF CONSCIOUSNESS

Karmic traces remain with us as psychic remnants of actions performed with grasping or aversion. They are obscurations of consciousness stored in the base consciousness of the individual, in the *kunzhi namshe**. Although it is spoken of as a container, the kunzhi namshe actually is equivalent to the obscuration of consciousness: when there are no obscurations of consciousness there is no kunzhi namshe. It is not a thing or a place; it is the dynamic that underlies the organization of dualistic experience. It is as insubstantial as a collection of habits, and as powerful as the habits that allow language to make sense, forms to resolve into objects, and existence to appear to us as something meaningful that we can navigate and understand.

The common metaphor for the kunzhi namshe is of a storehouse or repository that cannot be destroyed. We can think of the kunzhi namshe storing a collection of patterns or schematics. It is a grammar of experience that is affected to a greater or lesser extent by each action that we take externally or internally, physically or cognitively. As long as habitual tendencies exist in the mind of the individual, the kunzhi namshe exists. When one dies and the body deteriorates, the kunzhi namshe does not. The karmic traces continue in the mental consciousness until they are purified. When they are completely purified, there is no longer a kunzhi namshe and the individual is a buddha.

KARMIC TRACES AND DREAM

All samsaric experience is shaped by karmic traces. Moods, thoughts, emotions, mental images, perceptions, instinctive reactions, "common sense," and even our sense of identity are all governed by the workings of karma. For example, you may wake up feeling depressed. You have breakfast, everything seems to be all right, but there is a sense of depression that cannot be accounted for. We say in this case that some karma is ripening. The causes and conditions have come together in such a way that the depression manifests. There may be a hundred reasons for this depression to occur on this particular morning, and it may manifest in a myriad of ways. It may also manifest during the night as a dream.

In dream, the karmic traces manifest in consciousness unfettered by the rational mind with which we so often rationalize away a feeling or a fleeting mental image. We can think of the process like this: during the day the consciousness illuminates the senses and we experience the world, weaving sensory and psychic experiences into the meaningful whole of our life. At night the consciousness withdraws from the senses and resides in the base. If we have developed a strong practice of presence with much experience of the empty, luminous nature of mind, then we will be aware of and in this pure, lucid awareness. But for most of us the consciousness illuminates the obscurations, the karmic traces, and these manifest as a dream.

The karmic traces are like photographs that we take of each experience. Any reaction of grasping or aversion to any experience—to memories, feelings, sense perceptions, or thoughts—is like snapping a photo. In the darkroom of our sleep we develop the film. Which images are developed on a particular night will be determined by the secondary conditions recently encountered. Some images or traces are burned deeply into us by powerful reactions while others, resulting from superficial experiences, leave only a faint residue. Our consciousness, like the light of a projector, illuminates the traces that have been stimulated and they manifest as the images and experiences of the dream. We string them together like a film, as this is the way our psyches work to make meaning, resulting in a narrative constructed from conditioned tendencies and habitual identities: the dream.

This same process continually occurs while we are awake, making up what we commonly think of as "our experience." The dynamics are easier to understand in dream, because they can be observed free of the limitations of the physical world and the rational consciousness. During the day, although still engaged in the same dream-making process, we project this inner activity of the mind onto the world and think that our experiences are "real" and external to our own mind.

In dream yoga, this understanding of karma is used to train the mind to react differently to experience, resulting in new karmic traces from which are generated dreams more conducive to spiritual practice. It is not about force, about the consciousness acting imperially to oppress the unconscious. Dream yoga relies instead upon increased awareness and insight to allow us to make positive choices in life. Understanding the dynamic structure of experience and the consequences of actions leads to the recognition that every experience of any kind is an opportunity for spiritual practice.

Dream practice also gives us a method of burning the seeds of future karma during the dream. If we abide in awareness during a dream, we can allow the karmic traces to self-liberate as they arise and they will not continue on to manifest in our life as negative states. As in waking life, this will only happen if we can remain in the non-dual awareness of *rigpa**, the clear light of the mind. If this is not possible for us, we can still develop tendencies to choose spiritually positive behavior even in our dreams until we can go beyond preferences and dualism altogether.

Ultimately, when we purify the obscurations until none remain, there is no film, no hidden karmic influences that color and shape the light of our consciousness. Because karmic traces are the roots of dreams, when they are entirely exhausted only the pure light of awareness remains: no movie, no story, no dreamer and no dream, only the luminous fundamental nature that is absolute reality. This is why enlightenment is the end of dreams and is known as "awakening."

THE SIX REALMS OF CYCLIC EXISTENCE

According to the teachings, there are six realms (*loka**) of existence* in which all deluded beings exist. These are the realms of gods, demi-gods, humans, animals, hungry ghosts, and hell-beings. Fundamentally, the realms are six dimensions of consciousness, six dimensions of possible experience. They manifest in us indivdually as the six negative emotions: anger, greed, ignorance, jealousy, pride, and pleasurable distraction. (Pleasurable distraction is the emotional state when the other five emotions are present in equal measure, harmoniously balanced.) The six realms are not, however, only categories of emotional experience but are also actual realms into which beings are born, just as we were born into the human realm or a lion is born into the animal realm.

Each realm can be thought of as a continuum of experience. The hell realm, for instance, ranges from the internal emotional experience of anger and hatred, to behaviors rooted in anger such as fighting and wars, to institutions, prejudices, and biases built on hatred such as armies, racial hatred, and intolerance, to the actual realm in which beings exist. A name for the entirety of this dimension of experience, from individual emotion to actual realm, is "hell."

Like dreams, the realms are manifestations of karmic traces, but in the instance of the realms, the karmic traces are collective rather than individual. Because the karma is collective, the beings in each realm share similar experiences in a consensual world, as we share similar experiences with other humans. Collective karma creates bodies and senses and mental capacities that allow individuals to participate in shared potentials and categories of experience while making other kinds of experience impossible. Dogs, for example, can collectively hear sounds that humans cannot, and humans experience language in a way that dogs cannot.

Although the realms appear to be distinct and solid, as our world seems to us, they are actually dreamy and insubstantial. They interpenetrate one another and we are connected to each. We have the seeds of rebirth into the other realms in us, and when we experience different emotions we participate in some of the characteristic qualities and suffering predominant in other realms. When we are caught up in self-centered pride or angry envy, for example, we experience something of the characteristic quality of experience of the demi-god realm.

Sometimes individuals have a predominance of one dimension in their makeup: more animal, or more hungry ghost, or more god nature, or more demi-god. It stands out as the dominant trait of their character, and can be recognized in the way they talk, in their walk, and in their relationships. We may know people who always seem to be trapped in the hungry ghost realm: they can never get enough, they are always hungry for more of everything—more from their friends, their environment, their life—but can never be satisfied. Or perhaps we know someone who seems like a hell being: angry, violent, raging, in turmoil. More commonly, people have aspects of all the dimensions in their individual make-ups.

As these dimensions of consciousness manifest in emotions, it becomes apparent how universal they are. For example, every culture knows jealousy. The appearance of jealousy may vary because emotional expression is a means of communication, a language of gesture, determined both by biology and culture, and culture provides the variable. But the feeling of jealousy is the same everywhere. In Bön-Buddhism, this universality is explained by and correlated with the reality of the realms.

The six negative emotions are not meant to constitute an exhaustive list of emotions. It is pointless to argue about where sadness or fear fits into the realms. Fear can occur in any of the realms as can sadness or anger or jealousy or love. Although the negative emotions are affective experiences that we have, and are characteristic affective experiences of the realms, they are also keywords representing the entire dimension of experience, the continuum from individual emotional experience to actual realms. And those dimensions each encompass wide possiblities of experience, including diverse emotional experience.

The six qualities of consciousness are called paths because they lead somewhere: they take us to the places of our rebirth as well as into different realms of experience in this life. When a being identifies with, or is ensnared by, one of the negative emotions, certain results occur. This is the way karma actually works. For example, in order to be born as a human, we must have been heavily involved in moral disciplines in previous lifetimes. Even in popular culture this is expressed in the observation that it is not until love and concern for others matures that a person is considered to be "fully human."

If we live a life characterized by the negative emotions of hatred or anger, we experience a different result: we are reborn in hell. This happens actually, that a being may be born in the hell realm, as well as psychologically. Connecting oneself to the dimension of hatred produces experiences that even in this life we call hellish.

Clearly this does not mean that all humans try to avoid these experiences. Karma may lead a person so strongly into a dimension of experience that the negative emotion becomes attractive. Think of all the "entertainment" full of hatred, killing, and war. We can develop a taste for it. We say "War is hell," yet many of us are drawn to war.

Our bias toward one or another of these dimensions can also be shaped by the culture. For instance, in a society in which the angry warrior is considered heroic, we may be led in that direction. This is an example of the cultural ignorance described previously.

Although the realms may sound fanciful to people in the West, the manifestation of the six realms can be recognized in our own experience, in our dreams and waking lives, and in the lives of people near us. Sometimes, for example, we may feel lost. We know how to go about our daily routine, but the significance eludes us. The meaning is gone, not through liberation, but through lack of understanding. We have dreams of being in mud, or a in dark place, or on a street with no signs. We arrive in a room that has no exit, or feel confusion about which direction to take. This may be a manifestation of ignorance, the animal realm. (This ignorance is not the same as the innate ignorance. Instead it is a dullness, a lack of intelligence.)

We experience something of the god realm when we are lost in pleasurable distraction, enjoying hazy periods of pleasure and happiness. But these periods eventually come to an end. And while they last, our awareness must be constricted. We must remain in a kind of superficiality and avoid looking too deeply into the situation around us, avoid becoming aware of the suffering around us. It is good to enjoy pleasant periods in our lives, but if we do not practice, do not continue to free ourselves of constricting and erroneous identities, eventually we will pass through the period of pleasantness and fall into a more difficult state, unprepared, where we are likely to be lost in some kind of suffering. At the end of a party or a very pleasant day there is often a kind of letdown or depression upon returning home. Or after a happy weekend we may feel disappointed when we return to work.

We all have periods during which we experience different realms: the happiness of the god realm, maybe while we're on vacation or on a walk with friends, the ache of greed when we see something we feel we must have, the shame of wounded pride, the pangs of jealousy, the hellishness of bitterness and hatred, the dullness and confusion of ignorance. We move from the experience of one realm to another easily and frequently. We have all had the experience of being in a happy mood, connected to the god realm; the sun is out, people appear beautiful, we feel good about ourselves. Then we receive bad news or a friend says something that hurts us. Suddenly the world itself appears to have changed. Laughter sounds hollow, the sky is cold and uncaring, we no longer find others attractive nor do we enjoy ourselves. We have changed dimensions of experience and the world seems to have changed with us. Just so, do beings in other realms remain connected to all the realms; both a cat and a demi-god may experience anger, jealousy, emotional hunger, and so on.

During our dreaming lives, too, we experience the six realms. Just as the six negative emotions determine the quality of experience during the day, they shape the feeling and content of dreams. Dreams are of infinite variety but all karmic dreams are connected to one or more of the six dimensions.

Below is a brief description of the six realms. Traditionally, the realms are presented as descriptions of places and the beings that inhabit those places. The hells, for example, are eighteen in number, nine hot and nine cold hells. All the details in the traditional descriptions have meaning, but here we are focused on the experiences of the realms right now, in this life. We connect to each dimension of experience energetically through an energy center (*chakra**) in the body. The locations are listed below. The chakras are important in many different practices and play an important role in dream yoga.

Hell Realm

Anger is the seed emotion of the hell realm. When the karmic traces of anger manifest, there are many possible expressions, such as aversion, tension, resentment, criticism, argument, and violence. Much of the destruction of wars is caused by anger, and many people die every

REALM	PRIMARY EMOTION	CHAKRA
God (Devas)	Pleasurable distraction	Crown
Demi-god (Asuras)	Envy	Throat
Human	Jealousy	Heart
Animal	Ignorance	Navel
Hungry-ghost (Pretas)	Greed	Sexual Organs
Hell	Hatred	Soles of the feet

day as a result of anger. Yet anger never resolves any problem. When anger overcomes us we lose control and self-awareness. When we are trapped or victimized by hatred, violence, and anger, we are participating in the hell realm.

The energetic center of anger is in the soles of the feet. The antidote for anger is pure unconditioned love, which arises from the unconditioned self.

Traditionally, the hells are said to be composed of nine hot hells and nine cold hells. The beings who live there suffer immeasurably, being tortured to death and instantly returning to life, time after time.

Hungry Ghost Realm

Greed is the seed emotion of the hungry ghost (*preta*) realm. Greed arises as a feeling of excessive need that cannot be fulfilled. The attempt to satisfy greed is like drinking salty water when thirsty. When lost in greed we look outward rather than inward for satisfaction, yet we never find enough to fill the emptiness we wish to escape. The real hunger we feel is for knowledge of our true nature.

Greed is associated with sexual desire; its energetic center in the body is the chakra behind the genitals. Generosity, the open giving of what others need, unties the hard knot of greed.

The pretas are traditionally represented as beings with huge, hungry bellies and tiny mouths and throats. Some inhabit parched lands where there is not even a mention of water for hundreds of years. Others may find food and drink, yet if they swallow even a little through their tiny mouths, the food bursts into flame in their stomachs and causes great pain. There are many kinds of suffering for pretas, but all result from stinginess and opposing the generosity of others.

Animal Realm

Ignorance is the seed of the animal realm. It is experienced as a feeling of being lost, dull, uncertain, or unaware. Many people experience a darkness and sadness rooted in this ignorance; they feel a need but do not even know what they want or what to do to satisfy themselves. In the West, people are often considered happy if they are continually busy, yet we can be lost in ignorance in the midst of our busyness when we do not know our true nature.

The chakra associated with ignorance is in the center of the body at the level of the navel. The wisdom found when we turn inward and come to know our true self is the antidote to ignorance.

Beings in the animal realm are dominated by the darkness of ignorance. Animals live in fear because of the constant threat from other animals and humans. Even large animals are tormented by insects that burrow into their skin and live on their flesh. Domesticated animals are milked, loaded down, castrated, pierced through the nose, and ridden, without being able to escape. Animals feel pain and pleasure, but they are dominated by the ignorance that prevents them from looking beneath the circumstances of their lives to find their true nature.

Human Realm

Jealousy is the root emotion of the human realm. When possessed by jealousy, we want to hold on to and draw to ourselves what we have: an idea, a possession, a relationship. We see the source of happiness as something external to us, which leads to greater attachment to the object of our desire.

Jealousy is related to the heart center in the body. The antidote to jealousy is great openness of the heart, the openness that arises when we connect to our true nature.

It is easy for us to observe the suffering of our own realm. We experience birth, sickness, old age, and death. We are plagued by loss due to constant change. When we attain the object of our desire, we struggle to keep it, but its eventual loss is certain. Rather than rejoicing in the happiness of others, we often fall prey to envy and jealousy. Even though human birth is considered the greatest of good fortune because humans have the chance to hear and practice the teachings, only a tiny minority of us ever find our way to, and avail ourselves of, this great opportunity.

Demi-god Realm

Pride is the principal affliction of the demi-gods (*asuras*). Pride is a feeling connected to accomplishment and is often territorial. One cause of war is the pride of individuals and nations that believe they have the solution to other people's problems. There is a hidden aspect of pride that manifests when we believe ourselves worse than others in a particular ability or trait, a negative self-centeredness that singles us out from others.

Pride is associated with the chakra in the throat. Pride is often manifested in wrathful action, and its antidote is the great peace and humility that arises when we rest in our true nature.

The asuras enjoy pleasure and abundance but they tend toward envy and wrath. They continually fight with one another, but their greatest suffering occurs when they declare war on the gods, who enjoy even greater abundance than the demi-gods. The gods are more powerful than asuras and very difficult to kill. They always win the wars, and the asuras suffer the emotional devastation of wounded pride and envy in which they feel diminished and which, in turn, drives them into futile wars again and again.

God Realm

Pleasurable distraction is the seed of the god realm. In the god realm, the five negative emotions are equally present, balanced like five harmonious voices in a chorus. The gods are lost in a heady sense of lazy joy and self-centered pleasure. They enjoy great wealth and comfort in lives that last as long as an eon. All needs seem to be fulfilled and all desires sated. Just as is true for some individuals and societies, the gods become trapped in pleasure and the pursuit of pleasure. They have no sense of the reality beneath their experience. Lost in meaningless diversions and pleasures, they are distracted and do not turn to the path to liberation.

But the situation ultimately changes as the karmic causes for existence in the god realm are exhausted. As death finally approaches, the dying god is abandoned by friends and companions, who are unable to face the proof of their own mortality. The previously perfect body ages and deteriorates. The period of happiness is over. With divine eyes the god can see the conditions of the realm of suffering into which he or she is fated to be reborn, and even before death the suffering of that coming life begins.

The god realm is associated with the chakra at the crown of the head. The antidote to the selfish joy of the gods is encompassing compassion that arises spontaneously through awareness of the reality underlying self and world.

WHY "NEGATIVE" EMOTION?

Many people in the West are uncomfortable when they hear emotions labeled as negative, but it is not that emotions in themselves are negative. All emotions aid in survival and are necessary for the full range of human experience, including the emotions of attachment, anger, pride, jealousy, and so on. Without the emotions we would not live fully.

However, emotions are negative insofar as we become ensnared in them and lose touch with the deeper aspects of ourselves. They are negative if we react to them with grasping or aversion, because we then suffer a constriction of consciousness and identity. We then sow the seeds of future negative conditions that trap us in realms of suffering, both in this life and in subsequent lives, where it may be difficult to undertake the spiritual journey. And this result is negative when compared to a more expansive identity and particularly when compared to liberation from all contrived and constricted identities. This is why it is important to think of the realms not just as emotions but as six dimensions of consciousness and experience.

There are cultural differences regarding emotion. For example, fear and sadness are not often mentioned in the teachings, yet most of samsara is tinged with both. And the concept of self-hatred is alien to Tibetans, who do not have words to describe it. When I went to Finland, many people talked to me about depression; this was in sharp contrast to Italy, where I had just been and where people seem to talk about depression very little. The climate, religion, traditions, and spiritual belief systems condition us and affect our experience. But the underlying mechanism of how we are stuck—the grasping and aversion, the projection, and the dualistic interaction with what we project—is the same everywhere. This is what is negative in emotional experience.

If we truly understood and experienced the empty nature of reality, there would be no grasping and therefore no grosser form of the emotion, but, ignorant of the true nature of phenomena, we grasp at projections of the mind as if they were real. We develop a dualistic relationship with illusions, feeling anger or greed or some other emotional reaction in relation to them. In absolute reality there is no separate entity that is the target of our anger, or the object of any emotion. There is no reason to get angry at all. We create the story, the projections, and the anger at the same time.

Often in the West, the understanding of emotions is used in psychology to try to improve people's lives in samsara. That is good. However, the Tibetan system has a different goal and is more intent on understanding emotions so that we might get free of the constrictions and erroneous views that we hold onto through emotional attachment. Again, this does not mean that emotions are negative in themselves, but that they are negative to the extent that we cling to them or flee from them.

3   The Energy Body

All experience, waking and dreaming, has an energetic basis. This vital energy is called *lung** in Tibetan, but is better known in the West by its Sanskrit name, *prana**. The underlying structure of any experience is a precise combination of various conditions and causes. If we are able to understand why and how an experience is occurring, and recognize its mental, physical, and energetic dynamics, then we can reproduce those experiences or alter them. This allows us to generate experiences that support spiritual practice and avoid those that are detrimental.

CHANNELS AND PRANA

In daily life we take different bodily positions without thinking of their effects. When we want to relax and talk with friends we go to a room that contains comfortable chairs or sofas. This increases the experience of calm and relaxation and is conducive to easy conversation. But when we are active in business discussions we go to an office where the chairs hold us more erect and less relaxed. This is more supportive of business and creative endeavors. If we want to rest in silence we might go to the porch and sit in still another kind of chair situated so that we can enjoy the landscape and the flow of the air. When we grow tired we go to the bedroom and take a completely different posture to induce sleep.

Similarly, we assume various postures in different types of meditation to alter the flow of prana in the body by manipulating the channels* (*tsa**), which are the conduits of energy in the body, and to open

different energetic focal points, the chakras. Doing this evokes different kinds of experience. It is also the basis for the movements of yoga.
Consciously guiding the energy in our body allows for an easier and
more rapid development of meditation practice than would occur if
we relied only on the mind. It also allows us to overcome certain obstacles in practice. Without using the knowledge of prana and its movement in the body, the mind can become mired in its own processes.

Channels, prana, and chakras are involved in death as well as life.
Most mystical experiences as well as experiences in the intermediate
state after death result from the opening and closing of energy points.
Many books reporting on the phenomena of near-death experiences
contain descriptions of various lights and visions that people experience as they begin the death process. According to the Tibetan tradition, these phenomena have to do with the movement of prana. The
channels are associated with different elements; during the dissolution of the elements at death, as the channels deteriorate, the released
energy manifests in experience as light and color. The teachings go
into great detail about which colored light corresponds to the dissolution of which channel, where it is in the body, and to which emotion it
is related.

There is considerable variation in how these lights appear to people
at death, because they are related to both the negative emotional and
positive wisdom aspects of consciousness. The average person experiences emotions at death, and the dominant emotion determines the
lights and colors that manifest. Often there is, at first, only an experience of colored lights in which one color is primary, but it may also be
the case that a few colors are predominant or that there is a combination of many colors. The light then begins to form different images, as
it does in dream: of houses, castles, mandalas, people, deities, or almost anything else. When we are dying, we may relate to such visions
as either samsaric entities, in which case we are governed by our reactions to them in moving toward our next birth, or as meditative experiences, which allows us the opportunity of liberation or at least the possibility of consciously influencing our next birth in a positive direction.

CHANNELS (TSA)

There are many different kinds of channels in the body. We know of
the grosser channels through the medical study of anatomy, from which
we learn about blood vessels, the circulation of lymph, the network of
nerves, and so on. There are also channels, such as those recognized

in acupuncture, that are conduits for the more substantive forms of prana. In dream yoga we are concerned with an even subtler psychic energy that underlies both wisdom and negative emotion. The channels that carry this very subtle energy cannot be located in the physical dimension but we can become aware of them.

There are three root channels. Six major chakras are located on and in them. From the six chakras, three hundred and sixty branch channels spread throughout the body. The three root channels are, in women, the red channel on the right side of the body, the white channel on the left, and the blue central channel. In men, the right channel is white and the left channel is red. The three root channels join about four inches below the navel. The two side channels, which are the diameter of a pencil, rise up either side and in front of the spine and through the brain, curl under the skull at the top of the head, and open at the nostrils. The central channel rises straight up between them, in front of the spine. It is the diameter of a cane and widens slightly from the heart area to the crown of the head, where it ends.

The white channel (the right in men and the left in women) is the channel through which energies of the negative emotions move. Sometimes the channel is known as the channel of method. The red channel (the left in men, the right in women) is the conduit for positive or wisdom energies. Therefore, in dream practice, men sleep on their right side and women on their left in order to put pressure on the white channel and thus close it slightly while opening the red wisdom channel. This contributes to better experiences of dream, involving a more positive emotional experience and greater clarity.

The blue central channel is the channel of non-duality. It is in the central channel that the energy of primordial awareness (rigpa) moves. Dream practice ultimately brings the consciousness and the prana into the central channel, where it is beyond both negative and positive experience. When this occurs, the practitioner realizes the unity of all apparent dualities. Generally when people have mystical experiences, great experiences of bliss or emptiness or clarity or rigpa, they are energetically based in the central channel.

PRANA (LUNG)

Dreaming is a dynamic process. Unlike the static images of film that we use as a metaphor, the images of a dream are fluid: they move, beings talk, sounds vibrate, sensation is vivid. The content of dream is formed by the mind, but the basis of the vitality and animation of the dream is the prana. The literal translation of the Tibetan word for prana, lung, is "wind," but it is more descriptive to call it the vital wind force.

Prana is the foundational energy of all experience, of all life. In the East, people practice yoga positions and various breathing exercises to strengthen and refine the vital wind force in order to balance the body and the mind. Some of the ancient Tibetan esoteric teachings describe two different kinds of prana: karmic prana and wisdom prana.

Karmic Prana

Karmic prana is the energetic basis of the karmic traces produced as a result of all positive, negative, and neutral actions. When the karmic traces are activated by the appropriate secondary causes, karmic prana energizes them and allows them to have an effect in the mind, body, and dreams. Karmic prana is the vitality of both the negative and positive energies in both side channels.

When the mind is unstable, distracted, or unfocused, the karmic prana moves. This means, for example, when an emotion arises and the mind has no control over it, the karmic prana carries the mind wherever it will. Our attention moves here and there, pushed and pulled by aversion and desire.

Developing mental stability is necessary on the spiritual path, to make the mind strong, present, and focused. Then, even when the forces of the negative emotions arise, we are not blown into distraction by the karmic winds. In dream yoga, once we have developed the ability to have lucid dreams, we must be stable enough in presence to stabilize the dreams produced by the movement of the karmic prana and to develop control over the dream. Until the practice is developed, the dreamer will sometimes control the dream and sometimes the dream will control the dreamer.

Although some Western psychologies believe that the dreamer should not control the dream, according to Tibetan teachings this is a wrong view. It is better for the lucid and aware dreamer to control the dream than for the dreamer to be dreamed. The same is true with thoughts: it is better for the thinker to control the thoughts than for the thoughts to control the thinker.

Three Kinds of Karmic Prana

Some Tibetan yoga texts describe three kinds of karmic prana: soft prana, rough prana, and neutral prana. Soft prana refers to virtuous wisdom prana, which moves through the red wisdom channel. Rough prana refers to the prana of negative emotion, which moves through the white channel. In this classification, both virtuous wisdom prana and emotional prana are karmic prana.

Neutral prana is, as its name suggests, neither virtuous nor non-virtuous, but it is still karmic prana. It pervades the body. Experience of neutral prana leads the practitioner toward experience of the natural primordial prana, which is not karmic prana but the energy of nondual rigpa residing in the central channel.

Wisdom Prana

The wisdom prana (*ye lung*), is not karmic prana. It is not to be confused with the virtuous wisdom karma described in the section above.

In the first moment of any experience, before a reaction occurs, there is only pure perception. The prana involved in this pure experiencing is the primordial wisdom prana, the energy that underlies experience prior to or free of grasping or aversion. This pure experience does not leave a trace and is not the cause of any dream. The wisdom prana moves in the central channel and is the energy of rigpa. This moment is very brief, a flash of pure experience of which we are usually unaware. It is our reaction to this moment, our grasping and aversion, that we think of as our experience.

Pranic Activity

The Tibetan teacher Long-chen-pa says in one text that there are 21,600 movements of prana during a single day. Whether taken literally or not, the statement indicates the enormous activity of prana and thought occurring each day.

BALANCING THE PRANA

This is a simple practice one can do to balance the prana: Men should use the left ring finger to close the left nostril and exhale strongly from the right nostril. Imagine that all stress and negative emotions flow out with the exhalation. Then close the right nostril with the right ring finger and inhale deeply, very softly and gently, through the left nostril. After inhaling let all the air, the prana, pervade your entire body while you hold the breath for a short period. Then gently exhale and remain in a calm state.

Women reverse the order. Begin by closing the right nostril with the right ring finger and exhale sharply from the left nostril, emptying the lungs. Then close the left nostril with the left ring finger and gently and deeply inhale through the right nostril, breathing in the calm wisdom prana. Remain with calm pervading your body. Then gently exhale and remain in a calm state.

Repeating this again and again will balance one's energy. The rough emotional prana is exhaled from the white channel and the blissful wisdom prana is inhaled through the red channel. Allow the neutral prana to pervade the entire body. Abide in that calm.

PRANA AND MIND

All dreams are related to one or more of the six realms. The energetic connection between the mind and the realm is made through specific locations in the body. How can this be? We say that consciousness is beyond shape, color, time, or touch, so how can it be connected to place? The fundamental mind is beyond any such distinctions, but the qualities that arise in consciousness are influenced by the phenomena of experience.

We can look into this question for ourselves. Go somewhere peaceful, a beautiful temple filled with gentle singing and the smell of incense, or the green grotto of a small waterfall. When we enter such a place, it is as if a blessing is received. The quality of experience is affected because the physical environment affects the state of consciousness. This is also true for negative influences. When visiting a location that has been the site of atrocities we become uneasy; we say the place has "bad energy."

The same is true internally, inside our bodies. When we talk about bringing the mind to a chakra, to the heart chakra for example, what do we mean? What does it mean for the mind to be somewhere? Mind is not something that can be localized in the sense that it can be contained in a small area. When we "put" the mind somewhere we are

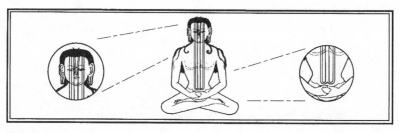

The Channels

placing our attention: we are creating images in our mind or directing attention to a sense object. When we focus the mind on something, the object of focus affects the quality of consciousness and there are correlated changes in the body.

This principle underlies healing practices that make use of mental imagery. Visualization leads to changes in our bodies. Western research is demonstrating the truth of this statement, and Western medicine is now using the power of visualization even for serious illnesses such as cancer. The Bön tradition of healing often uses visualization of the elements: fire, water, and wind. Rather than addressing the symptoms of the disease, the follower of Bön generally attempts to purify the underlying conditioning of the mind, the negative emotions and karmic traces that are believed to create susceptibility to disease.

For example, we may visualize intense fire in response to an illness. We visualize red triangular shapes and try to imaginatively experience heat—as powerful as that rising from a volcano—moving through our bodies like waves of flame. We may do a particular breathing exercise to generate even more heat. In this way, we use the mind and its images to affect the body, the emotions, and the energy. And there is a result even though we have thrown no switch in the external world. Just as Western medicine may use radiation therapy to attempt to burn cancer cells, we use internal fire to burn up the karmic traces. In order for the practice to be effective, the intention must be clear as well. It is not a simple mechanical process, but one that uses the understanding of karma, mind, and prana to aid in healing. This practice has the advantage of attempting to resolve the cause of the disease rather than the symptoms, and of being free of side effects. Of course, it is good also to avail ourselves of Western medicine when possible. Rather than limit ourselves to a particular system, it is better to use whatever is beneficial.

CHAKRAS

In dream practice, we direct our attention into different areas in the body: the chakras at the throat, brow, and heart, and the secret chakra, behind the genitals. A chakra is a wheel of energy, a nexus of energetic connections. Channels of energy meet at particular locations in the body; the junctions of the channels form the energetic patterns that are chakras. The major chakras are sites where many channels join.

Chakras are not really like the pictures drawn of them, of lotuses that open and close, that have a certain number of petals and a certain color. Such images are only symbolic supports for the mind—like maps—that we use to help focus the attention on the patterns of energy that exist at the site of the chakras. The chakras were initially discovered through practice, through the realizations of different practitioners. When these practitioners initially developed experiences of the chakras, there was no language that could describe their discoveries to those who had not had the same experience. Images were created that could be used as visual metaphors and to which other people could relate. The various images of the lotus, for instance, suggested that the energy around a chakra expanded and contracted like the opening and closing of a flower; one chakra felt different from another and these differences were represented by different colors; experiences of varying concentrations and complexities of energy in the different chakras were represented by different numbers of petals. These visual metaphors became the language used to articulate the experiences of the energy centers in the body. When a new practitioner visualizes the right number of petals at the right spot in the body, with the right color, then the power of the mind affects that particular energetic point and is influenced by that point. When this occurs, we say that mind and prana are unified in the chakra.

BLIND HORSE, LAME RIDER

At night, when we go to sleep, we generally do so with little sense of what is happening. We just feel tired, shut our eyes, and drift away. We may have an idea about sleep—blood in the brain, hormones, or something like that—but the actual process of falling asleep remains mysterious and unexplored.

The Tibetan tradition explains the process of falling asleep using a metaphor for the mind and prana. Often prana is compared to a blind horse and the mind to a person unable to walk. Separately they are helpless, but together they make a functional unit. When the horse and rider are together they begin to run, generally with little control over where they go. We know this from our own experience: we can "put" the mind into a chakra by placing attention there, but it is not easy to keep the mind in any one place. The mind is always moving, our attention going to this or that. Normally, in samsaric beings, the horse and rider run blindly through one of the six dimensions of consciousness, one of the six negative emotional states.

For example, as we fall asleep, awareness of the sensory world is lost. The mind is carried here and there on the blind horse of karmic prana until it becomes focused in a particular chakra where it is influenced by a particular dimension of consciousness. Perhaps you had an argument with your partner and that situation (secondary condition) activates a karmic trace associated with the heart chakra, which pulls your mind into that location in the body. The subsequent activity of mind and prana manifests in the particular images and stories of the dream.

The mind is not driven randomly to one chakra or another, but rather is drawn to the places in the body and the situations in life that need attention and healing. In the example, it is as if the heart chakra is crying out for help. The disturbing trace will be healed by manifesting in the dream and thereby being exhausted. However, unless the manifestation takes place while the dreamer is centered and aware, the reactions to it will be dictated by habitual karmic tendencies and will create more karmic seeds.

We can think of a computer as an analogy. The chakras are like different files. Click on the directory "Prana and Mind," and then open the file of the heart chakra. The information in the file—the karmic traces associated with the heart chakra—is displayed on the screen of awareness. This is like the dream manifesting.

Then perhaps a situation in the dream elicits another response that energizes a different emotion. The dream now becomes the secondary cause that allows another karmic trace to manifest. Now the mind travels down to the navel center and enters a different realm of experience. The character of the dream changes. You are not jealous anymore; instead you are on a street without signs or somewhere very dark. You are lost. You try to go somewhere but you cannot find your way. You are in the animal realm, the dimension most connected to ignorance.

Basically, this is how the content of the dream is shaped. The mind and prana are drawn to different chakras in the body; affected by the associated karmic traces, experiences of the various dimensions of experience arise in the mind as the character and content of the dream. We can use this understanding to look at our dreams differently, to notice which emotion and realm is connected to the dream. It is also helpful to understand that every dream offers us an opportunity for healing and spiritual practice.

Ultimately, we wish to stabilize the mind and the prana in the central channel rather than allowing the mind to be drawn to a particular chakra. The central channel is the energetic basis of experiences of rigpa, and the practices that we do in dream yoga are meant to bring mind and prana into the central channel. When this occurs, we remain in clear awareness and strong presence. To dream in the central channel is to dream free of strong influences from the negative emotions. It is a balanced situation that allows dreams of knowledge and clarity to manifest.

4 Summary: How Dreams Arise

Prior to realization, the individual's true nature is obscured by the root ignorance that gives rise to the conceptual mind. Ensnared in dualistic vision, the conceptual mind divides the seamless unity of experience into conceptual entities and then relates to these mental projections as if they inherently exist as separate beings and things. The primary dualism divides experience into self and other, and from the identification with only one aspect of experience, the self, preferences develop. This results in the arising of aversion and desire, which become the basis for both physical and mental actions. These actions (karmas) leave traces in the individual's mind as conditioned tendencies, resulting in more grasping and aversion, which lead to new karmic traces, and so on. This is the self-perpetuating cycle of karma.

During sleep the mind is withdrawn from the sensory world. Karmic traces currently stimulated by secondary causes necessary for their manifestation have a force or energy that is the karmic prana. Like the horse and rider in the analogy, the mind "rides" the karmic prana to the energetic center in the body related to the activated karmic trace. That is, the consciousness becomes focused in a particular chakra.

In this interplay of mind, energy, and meaning, consciousness illuminates and is affected by the karmic traces and the qualities of the associated realm. The karmic prana is the energy of the dream, the vital force, while the mind weaves the specific manifestations of the karmic traces—the color, light, emotions, and images—into the meaningful story that is the dream. This is the process that results in the samsaric dream.

5   Images from the *Mother Tantra*

In the Great Perfection (Dzogchen) teachings, the issue is always whether or not we recognize our true nature and understand that the reflections of that nature manifest as experience. The dream is a reflection of our own mind. This is easy to believe after we wake up, just as the Buddhas know—after they are enlightened—that the entities and objects of samsara are illusory. And just as it takes practice to recognize the illusory nature of dream while asleep, we must practice to realize the illusory nature of waking life. With some understanding of how dreams arise, it may be easier to understand what is meant by "illusory" and "lacking inherent existence," and also, importantly, easier to apply this understanding to our experience. The process by which experience arises is the same whether we are dreaming or awake. The world is a dream, the teacher and the teaching are a dream, the result of our practice is a dream; there is no place where the dream breaks until we are liberated into pure rigpa. Until then, we continue to dream ourselves and our lives in both the dream and the physical dimension.

Not knowing how to work with thought means one is controlled by thoughts. Knowing how to work with thought means that thought is brought into awareness and used either for positive purposes and virtuous action or is liberated into its empty essence. This is how thought is utilized in the path. In the same way, we can bring delusion, suffering, and any experience whatsoever into the path. But to do so we must understand that the essence of all that arises is empty.

When we do, then every moment of life is free and all experience is spiritual practice: all sound is mantra, all form is pure emptiness, and all suffering is a teaching. This is what is meant by "transforming into the path."

Directly realizing that anger has no objective basis but is only a reflection of mind, like a dream, the knot of anger loosens and it is no longer binding. When we realize that what we fear as a snake is only a rope that we have misperceived, the power of its appearance is gone. Understanding that appearances are empty luminosity leads to the recognition that mind and experience are a unity.

There is a Tibetan word, *lhun drub*, that translates as "spontaneous perfection." It means that there is no producer producing anything. Everything is just as it is, spontaneously arising from the base as a perfect manifestation of emptiness and clarity. A crystal does not make light: its natural function is simply to radiate light. The mirror does not select a face to reflect: its nature is to reflect everything. When we understand that everything arising, including our conventional sense of self, is only a projection of mind, then we are free. Without this understanding, it is as if we take a mirage to be real, an echo to be a sound not our own. The sense of separation is strong and we become trapped in an illusory dualism.

The *Mother Tantra*, one of the most important of the Bön texts, offers us examples, similes, and metaphors that we can ponder in order to better understand this illusory nature of both dream and waking life.

Reflection. The dream is a projection of our own mind. It is not different from the mind, just as a ray of sunlight is not different from the light of the sun in the sky. Not knowing this, we engage the dream as if it were real, like a lion snarling at the face it sees reflected in water. In a dream, the sky is our mind, the mountain is our mind; the flowers, the chocolate that we eat, the other people, all are our own mind reflected back at us.

Lightning. In the night sky, lightning flashes. Suddenly the mountains are illuminated, each peak seemingly a separate object, but what we are really experiencing is a single flash of light being reflected back to our eyes. Just so, the seemingly separate objects in a dream are actually the single light of our mind, the light of rigpa.

Rainbow. Like a rainbow, the dream can be beautiful and alluring. But is has no substance; it is a display of light and depends on the perspective of the observer. If we chase it, we can never reach it; there is nothing there. The dream, like the rainbow, is a combination of conditions from which an illusion arises.

Moon. The dream is like a moon reflected in many different waters—in the pond, the well, the sea—and in many different windows in a town, and in many different crystals. The moon is not multiplying. There is only one moon, just as the many objects of a dream are of one essence.

Magic. A magician can make a single stone appear first as an elephant, then as a snake, then as a tiger. But these different objects are illusory, like the objects in a dream that are all made from the light of the mind.

Mirage. Due to secondary causes we may see a mirage in a desert, a shimmering city or a lake. But when we approach we find nothing there. When we investigate the images of a dream, they, like the mirage, are found to be substanceless illusions, the play of light.

Echo. If we make a loud sound where there are conditions for echos, a loud sound returns to us; a quiet sound returns a quiet sound; and a strange cry comes back to us as a strange cry. The sound we hear returning is the sound we made, just as the content of a dream appears to be independent of us but is only the projected content of our mind returning to us.

These examples stress the lack of inherent existence and the unity of experience and experiencer. In the sutra teachings we call this "emptiness," in tantra "illusion," and in Dzogchen "the single sphere." The self and the object of experience are not two things. The world within and without is our own manifestation. We all share the same world because we share the same collective karma. How we view the phenomena of experience determines the kinds of experience we have and how we react to experience. We believe in our vision of entities that possess inherent existence, that live as separate beings and things. When we believe that something is actually there, then it is! It has power to affect us. We make the world to which we respond.

When we cease to exist, the world we make dissolves, not the world that other people inhabit. Our perception and the way we view everything ceases with us. If we dissolve our conceptual mind, the underlying purity manifests spontaneously. When we know directly that there is no inherent existence either in our self or the world, then whatever arises in experience has no power over us. When the lion mistakes his reflection in the water for something real, he is startled and snarls; when he understands the illusory nature of the reflection, he does not react with fear. Lacking true understanding, we react to the illusory projections of our own mind with grasping and aversion and create karma. When we know the true empty nature, we are free.

TEACHING METAPHORS

The *Mother Tantra* says that the ignorance of ordinary sleep is like a dark room. Awareness is the flame of a lamp. When the lamp is lit, the darkness is dispelled and the room is illuminated.

Instruction through symbols and metaphors is the most powerful way to communicate spiritual teachings in language. But it is a use of language one must learn to understand. Often, I find that students encounter difficulties with metaphors, so I wanted to add this note about how best to work with metaphors and symbolic images.

Using language to evoke sensory experience is more useful in the teachings than are explanations confined to abstract and technical concepts. Though the real experience cannot be communicated easily in any language, images used in the teachings help when they are perceived by more than just the rational mind. These metaphors are to be experienced, as are the images in poetry. They are to mulled over, pondered, experimented with, and integrated into experience.

For instance, when we hear the word "fire," we may pay little attention. But dwelling on it, allowing the image to emerge from behind the word, we see fire, we know the heat. Because we all know fire as more than a conceptual abstraction—because we have all watched flame and felt the heat of it on our skin—the word evokes an imaginal sensual experience. A fire burns in our imagination.

If we say "lemon" and let the fruit emerge from the word, our mouths water, our tongues constrict from sourness. With "chocolate," we almost have the sweet taste. Language is symbolic. In order to be meaningful it calls on memory and sense and imagination. When metaphors and symbols are used in the teaching, it is best to allow them to affect us in this way. Do not just think the words "a flame in a dark place," or "a reflection in a mirror." Use your senses, your body, and your imagination to understand. We must go beyond the image, but it can point us in the right direction.

When we enter a house illuminated by a lamp we do not examine the lamp, the wick, and the oil. We just experience the luminosity of the room. Try to do the same with teaching metaphors. Our minds, trained to work with abstractions and logic, seize a metaphor and analyze it. We ask too much of the metaphor. We want to know how the lamp got in the room, how the flame gets lit, how the wind starts. We want to know what kind of mirror it is, what it is made of, what stands outside of the mirror to be reflected. Instead, let yourself dwell in the image; try to find the experience hidden in the word. There is darkness. A lamp is lit. We all know this experience with our bodies and senses. The darkness is replaced by luminosity that is clear, substanceless, directly known. A wind arises and the flame is blown out. We know what it feels like when light is overcome by darkness.

PART TWO

Kinds and Uses of Dreams

The goal of dream practice is liberation; our intent should be to realize what is beyond dreams altogether. But there are also relative uses of dream that can be beneficial in our everyday life. These include both using information that we glean from dreams and directly benefiting from experiences that we have in the dream. In the West, for example, the use of dreams in therapy is widespread and there are many accounts of artists and scientists using the creativity of dreams to benefit their work. Tibetans also rely on dreams in various ways. This section describes some of the relative uses of dreams.

1 Three Kinds of Dreams

There are three types of dream that form a progression in dream practice, although not an exact one: 1) ordinary samsaric dreams, 2) dreams
of clarity, and 3) clear light dreams. The first two types are distinguished
by the differences of their causes, and in either, the dreamer may be
either lucid or non-lucid. In clear light dreams, there is awareness, but
no subject-object dichotomy. Clear light dreams occur in non-dual
awareness.

SAMSARIC DREAMS

The dreams that most of us have most of the time are the samsaric
dreams that arise from karmic traces*. Meaning found in these dreams
is meaning that we project into them; it is imputed by the dreamer

Ordinary dreaming (Arises from personal karmic traces)	Non-lucid Lucid
Dreams of clarity (Arise from transpersonal karmic traces)	Non-lucid Lucid
Clear light dreams (Non-duality)	Lucid (beyond subject/object duality)

rather than being inherent in the dream. This is also the case with meaning in our waking life. This does not make meaningful dreams unimportant any more than it makes the meaning in our waking life unimportant. The process is similar to reading a book. A book is just marks on paper, but because we bring our sense of meaning to it we can take meaning from it. And the meaning of a book, like a dream, is subject to interpretation. Two people can read the same book and have entirely different experiences; one person may change her whole life based on the meaning she has found in the pages, while her friend may find the book only mildly interesting or not even that. The book has not changed. The meaning is projected onto the words by the reader, and then read back.

DREAMS OF CLARITY

As progress is made in dream practice, dreams become clearer and more detailed, and a larger part of each dream is remembered. This is a result of bringing greater awareness into the dream state. Beyond this increased awareness in ordinary dreams is a second kind of dream called the dream of clarity, which arises when the mind and the prana are balanced and the dreamer has developed the capacity to remain in non-personal presence. Unlike the samsaric dream, in which the mind is swept here and there by karmic prana, in the dream of clarity the dreamer is stable. Though images and information arise, they are based less on personal karmic traces and instead present knowledge available directly from consciousness below the level of the conventional self. This is analogous to the differences in the rough karmic prana of the white channel, which is connected to negative emotion, and the wisdom prana of the red channel. Just as they are both karmic prana— energies involved in experiences of dualism—but one is purer and less deluded than the other, so is the dream of clarity purer and less deluded than the samsaric dream. In the dream of clarity it is as if something is given to or found by the dreamer, as opposed to the samsaric dream in which meaning is projected from the dreamer onto the purity of fundamental experience.

Dreams of clarity may occasionally arise for anyone, but they are not common until the practice is developed and stable. For most of us, all dreams are samsaric dreams based on our daily lives and emotions. Even though we may have a dream about the teachings, or our teachers, or our practice, or buddhas, or *dakinis**, the dream is still likely to be a samsaric dream. If we are involved in practice with a teacher, then of course we will dream about these things. It is a positive sign to have these dreams because it means that we are engaged in the teachings, but the engagement itself is dualistic and therefore in the realm of samsara. There are better and worse aspects of samsara, and it is good to be fully engaged in practice and the teachings because that is the path to liberation. It is also good not to mistake samsaric dreams for dreams of clarity.

If we make the mistake of believing that samsaric dreams are offering us true guidance, then changing our lives daily, trying to follow the dictates of dreams, can become a full-time job. It is also a way to become stuck in personal drama, believing that all our dreams are messages from a higher, more spiritual source. It is not like that. We should pay close attention to dreams and develop some understanding of which ones have import and which are only the manifestation of the emotions, desires, fears, hopes, and fantasies of our daily life.

CLEAR LIGHT DREAMS

There is a third type of dream that occurs when one is far along the path, the clear light dream. It arises from the primordial prana in the central channel. The clear light is generally spoken of in the teachings about sleep yoga and indicates a state free from dream, thought, and image, but there is also a clear light dream in which the dreamer remains in the nature of mind. This is not an easy accomplishment; the practitioner must be very stable in non-dual awareness before the clear light dream arises. Gyalshen Milu Samleg, the author of important commentaries on the *Mother Tantra*, wrote that he practiced consistently for nine years before he began to have clear light dreams.

Developing the capacity for clear light dreams is similar to developing the capacity of abiding in the non-dual presence of rigpa during the day. In the beginning, rigpa and thought seem different, so that in the experience of rigpa there is no thought, and if thought arises we are distracted and lose rigpa. But when stability in rigpa is developed, thought simply arises and dissolves without in the least obscuring rigpa; the practitioner remains in non-dual awareness. These situations are similar to learning to play the drum and bell together in ritual practice: in the beginning we can only do one at a time. If we play the bell, we lose the rhythm of the drum, and vice versa. After we are stable we can play both at the same time.

The clear light dream is not the same as the dream of clarity, which, while arising from deep and relatively pure aspects of the mind and generated from positive karmic traces, still takes place in duality. The clear light dream, while emerging from the karmic traces of the past, does not result in dualistic experience. The practitioner does not re-constitute as an observing subject in relation to the dream as an object, nor as a subject in the world of the dream, but abides wholly inte-grated with non-dual rigpa.

The differences in the three kinds of dreams may seem subtle. Samsaric dream arises from the individual's karmic traces and emo-tions, and all content of the dream is formed by those traces and emo-tions. The dream of clarity includes more objective knowledge, which arises from collective karmic traces and is available to consciousness when it is not entangled in personal karmic traces. The consciousness is then not bound by space and time and personal history, and the dreamer can meet with real beings, receive teachings from real teach-ers, and find information helpful to others as well as to him or herself.

The clear light dream is not defined by the content of the dream, but is a clear light dream because there is no subjective dreamer or dream ego, nor any self in a dualistic relationship with the dream or the dream content. Although a dream arises, it is an activity of the mind that does not disturb the practitioner's stability in clear light.

2 Uses of Dreams

The greatest value of dreams is in the context of the spiritual journey. Most importantly, they may be used as a spiritual practice in themselves. They may also provide the experiences that motivate the dreamer to enter the spiritual path. Furthermore, they can be a means of determining whether or not the practice is being done correctly, how much progress is being made, and what needs attention.

As in the story I told in the preface, it is often the case that before giving a high teaching the teacher will wait for the student to have a dream indicating his or her readiness to receive the teaching. Other dreams may demonstrate that the student has accomplished a certain practice, and after hearing the dream the teacher may determine that it is time for the student to move on to another practice.

In the same way, if we pay attention to dreams we can gauge our own maturity in the practice. Sometimes in the waking state we think we are doing quite well but when we sleep we find that at least some part of us is still greatly confused or stuck in negativity. This should not be viewed as a discouragement. It is a benefit when different aspects of the mind manifest in dream and point out where we must work in order to progress. On the other hand, when practice becomes very strong, the results of the practice will manifest in dream and give us confidence in our efforts.

EXPERIENCE IN DREAM

Experience is very flexible in dream and we are free to do a great many things that we cannot when awake, including particular practices that facilitate our development. We can heal wounds in the psyche, emotional difficulties that we have not been able to overcome. We can remove energetic blocks that may be inhibiting the free circulation of energy in the body. And we can pierce obscurations in the mind by taking experience beyond conceptual boundaries and limitations.

Generally, these tasks are best accomplished after we develop the ability to remain lucid in dream. It is only mentioned here as a possibility; in the section on practice there is more detail about what to do in the dream once lucidity is attained.

GUIDANCE AND GUIDELINES

Most Tibetans—high spiritual masters and simple, ordinary people—consider dreams to be a potential source of both the most profound spiritual knowledge and of guidance for everyday life. Dreams are consulted to diagnose illness, for indications that practices of purification or clarification are needed, and for indications that relationships to deities and guardians need attention. Such use of dreams may be thought superstitious, but on a profound level dreams portray the state of the dreamer and the condition of his or her relationship to different energies. In the East, people recognize these energies and relate to them as guardians and protector spirits as well as physiological conditions and internal spiritual conditions. In the West, with its much younger study of dreams, these energies may be understood as incipient illnesses or deeply rooted complexes or archetypes.

Some Tibetans work with dreams throughout their lives, as a primary form of communication with deeper aspects of themselves and with other worlds. My mother was a good example of this. She was a practitioner and a very loving and kind woman. Often she told the whole family her dreams in the morning, when we were gathered to eat, and particularly when the dream had to do with her guardian and protector, Namthel Karpo.

Namthel is a guardian of the Northern part of Tibet, Hor, where my mother grew up. Although his practice was known throughout Tibet, he was primarily worshiped in the village in which she lived and in the surrounding area. My mother did his practice, but my father did not, and often he would tease her after she recounted her dreams.

I clearly remember my mother telling us one dream in which Namthel came to her. He was dressed, as always, in white robes and

conch shell earrings, and he had long hair. This time he looked furi-
ous. He came through the door and roughly threw a little bag on the
floor. He said, "I always tell you to take care of yourself but you don't
do a good job of it!" He looked deeply into my mother's eyes and then
disappeared.

In the morning my mother was uncertain as to the dream's meaning. But in the afternoon a lady who sometimes worked in our home
tried to steal our money. She was carrying it tucked under her clothes
but when she walked in front of my mother the money fell out, right
there. It was in a bag identical to the one that my mother had been
shown in the dream. My mother picked it up and inside was all of our
money, about to be stolen. She considered this event an activity of
protection on the part of her guardian and believed that Namthel
caused the bag to fall to the floor.

Namthel appeared in my mother's dreams throughout her life, always appearing in the same form. Though the messages he gave her
varied, they were generally dreams meant to help her in some way, to
protect her and guide her.

Until I was ten years old I was in a Christian school, after which my
parents took me out and I entered the Meri Monastery. One of the
monks, Gen Sengtuk, would sometimes tell me his dreams. I remember some of them quite clearly as they were very similar to my
mother's. He often dreamt of Sippe Gyalmo, one of the most important and ancient of the enlightened protectors of the Bön tradition.
The practice of Sippe Gyalmo is also practiced in the other Tibetan
Buddhist schools; in the Potala Palace in Tibet, there is a room that
houses her shrine. Gen Sengtuk's dreams of Sippe Gyalmo guided
him in his life and practice.

Sippe Gyalmo did not appear in his dreams as the ferocious being
that we see in paintings in temples and meditation rooms. Instead, he
saw her as a very old, gray-haired human woman, in a body that was
no longer straight, using a walking stick. Gen Sengtuk always met
Sippe Gyalmo in a vast desert in which she had a tent. No one else
lived there. The monk would read her expressions, whether her face
was happy or sad, or if there was anger in the way she moved. And
reading her this way he would somehow know what to do to heal
obstacles in his practice or to change certain things in his life in a more
positive direction. This is how she guided him through his dreams.

He kept a close connection to her through dreams and she appeared to him in a similar manner throughout his life. His experiences with her are good examples of dreams of clarity.

I was a little boy then, and I can clearly remember one day when, listening to the monk recounting one of his dreams, it suddenly struck me that it was as if he had a friend in a different place. I thought it would be nice to have some friends to play with in dreams, because during the day I could not play much, as the studies were very intensive and the teachers strict. That was the thought I had then. So, you see, our understanding of dream and dream practice, and our motivation to do the practice, can become deeper and mature as we grow.

DIVINATION

Many meditation masters, because of the stability of their meditation practice, are able to use dreams of clarity for divination. To do so, the dreamer must be able to free himself or herself from most of the personal karmic traces that normally shape the dream. Otherwise, information is not obtained from the dream but is projected onto the dream, as is normally the case with samsaric dreams. This use of dreams is considered, in the Bön tradition, to be one of several methods of shamanic divination and is quite common among Tibetans. It is not unusual for a student to ask his or her teacher for guidance regarding an undertaking or for direction in overcoming an obstacle, and often the teacher turns to dreams to find the answer for the student.

For example, when I was in Tibet I met a realized Tibetan woman named Khachod Wangmo. She was very powerful and a "treasure finder" (*terton*) who had rediscovered many hidden teachings. I asked her for knowledge of my future, a general question about obstacles I would encounter and so on. I asked her to have a dream of clarity for me.

Commonly in this situation, the dreamer asks for a possession of the person requesting the dream. I gave Khachod Wangmo the undershirt I was wearing. The shirt represented me energetically, and by focusing on it she was able to connect to me. She put it under her pillow that night, then slept and had a dream of clarity. In the morning she gave me a long explanation of what was to come in my life, things that I should avoid and things that I should do. It was clear and helpful guidance.

Sometimes a student asks whether or not a dream that tells us something about the future demonstrates that the future is fixed. In the Tibetan tradition, we believe that it is not. The causes of all things that can happen are already present, right now, because the consequences of the past are the seeds of future situations. The primary causes of any situation in the future are to be found in what has already occurred. But the secondary causes necessary for the manifestation of the karmic seeds are not fixed, they are circumstantial. That is why practice is effective, and why illness can be cured. If it were otherwise, it would make no sense to attempt anything, as nothing could be changed. If we have a dream about tomorrow, and tomorrow comes and everything happens just as it did in our dream, this does not mean the future is fixed and cannot be changed; it means we did not change it.

Imagine a strong karmic trace, imprinted with a strong emotion, that is a primary cause for a particular situation, and it is coming to fruition. That is, our lives may be providing the secondary causes necessary for the primary cause to manifest. In a dream of the future, the cause is present and the trace that is ripening toward manifestation conditions the dream, with the result that the dream is an imagining of the results. It is as if we go into a kitchen and there is a wonderful Italian cook there, and the smell of spices and cooking food, and the ingredients laid out on a table: we can almost imagine the dinner that is being prepared, almost see the results of the situation. This is like the dream. We may not be completely accurate, but we might get most of it right. And then, when we are served the dinner, it will merge with our expectations, the differences will blur, and it will be the dinner we expected even if it is not quite the same.

I remember an example of this from when I was young. It was a day called Diwali in India, traditionally celebrated with firecrackers. My friends and I did not have money to buy firecrackers, so we looked for ones that had been lit but had not exploded. We gathered them and then tried to relight them. I was very young, four or five years old. One of the firecrackers was a little wet, and I put it on a burning coal. I shut my eyes and blew on it and of course it exploded. For a moment I could not see anything except stars, and right then I remembered my dream of the night before. It was exactly the same, the whole experience. Of course, it would have been much more helpful if I had remembered the dream before rather than after the event! There are many cases like this, in which the causes of future situations are woven into a dream about a future that is likely to, but will not necessarily, unfold.

Sometimes in a dream the causes and results affecting other people can be known. When I was in Tibet, my teacher, Lopon Tenzin Namdak, had a dream and then told me it was very important that I do a particular practice connected with one of the guardians. I began to do the practice for many hours every day while I traveled, trying to influence whatever he had seen in his dream. A few days after his dream, I was a passenger in a truck traveling on a tiny road high in the mountains. The drivers in that part of Tibet are wild, nomadic people with little fear of death. Thirty of us were crowded into a big truck with a lot of heavy luggage when the tire hit a hole and the truck tipped over.

I got out and looked down. I was not particularly afraid. But then I saw that one small stone held the truck up, preventing it from sliding down into a valley, a drop so far that a stone tossed over the edge took what seemed to be a long while to reach bottom. Then my heart started to bang around in my chest! Then I felt the fear, noticing that one small stone was all that stood between us and death, that kept my life from ending as a short story.

When I saw what the situation was I thought, "That's it. That's why I had to do the practice of the guardian." That was what my teacher saw in his dream and why he told me to do the practice. A dream may not be very specific, but still can convey through the feeling and images of the dream that something is coming that needs to be remedied. This is one kind of benefit we can receive from working with our dreams.

TEACHINGS IN DREAM

There are numerous examples in the Tibetan tradition of practitioners who received teachings in dreams. Often the dreams come in sequence, each night's dream starting where the previous night's dream ends, and in this way transmitting entire, detailed teachings until a precise and appropriate point of completion is reached, at which point the dreams stop. Volumes of teachings have been "discovered" this way, including many of the practices that Tibetans have been doing for centuries. This is what we call "mind treasure" (*gong-ter**).

Imagine entering a cave and finding a volume of teachings hidden inside. This is finding in a physical space. Mind treasures are found in consciousness rather than in the physical world. Masters have been known to find these treasures both in dreams of clarity and when awake. In order to receive these kinds of teaching in a dream, the practitioner must have developed certain capacities, such as being able to stabilize in consciousness without identifying with the conventional self. The practitioner whose clarity is unobscured by karmic traces and samsaric dreams has access to the wisdom inherent in consciousness itself.

Authentic teachings discovered in dream do not come from the intellect. It is not like going to the library and doing research and then writing a book, using the intellect to collect and synthesize information as a scholar might. Although many good teachings come from the intellect, they are not considered mind treasures. The wisdom of the Buddhas is self-originated, rising from the depths of consciousness, complete in itself. This does not mean that mind treasure teachings will not resemble existing teachings, for they will. Furthermore, these teachings can be found in different cultures and in different historical periods, and can be similar even though they do not inform each other. Historians work to trace a teaching back in time in order to point out how it was influenced by a similar teaching, where the historical connection took place, and so on, and often they find such a link. But the underlying truth is that these teachings arise spontaneously from humans when they reach a certain point in their individual development. The teachings are inherent in the foundational wisdom that any culture can eventually access. They are not only Buddhist or Bön teachings; they are teachings for all humans.

If we have the karma to help other beings, the teachings from a dream may be of benefit to others. But it may also be the case, if we have karma with a lineage, for example, that the teachings discovered in a dream will be particularly for our own practice, perhaps as a specific remedy to overcome a particular obstacle.

3   The Discovery of Chöd Practice

Many masters have used dream as an important wisdom door through which they have discovered teachings, made connections to masters who are otherwise distant in time and space, and developed the capacity to help others. All of these are illustrated in the story of Tongjung Thuchen, a great master of Bön, who is believed to have lived in the eighth century. In a series of dreams he discovered the Bön practice of *chöd**, a visionary practice of cultivating generosity and cutting through attachment.

By the time Tongjung Thuchen was six years old he was already knowledgeable about the teachings. At twelve he was making long retreats and having remarkable dream experiences in which he discovered teachings and met and received teachings from other masters. Once when he was in a retreat and intensively doing the practice of Walsai, one of the most important tantric deities of Bön, he was summoned by his master. He left the retreat and journeyed to the house of one of his master's sponsors, where he went to sleep and had an amazing dream.

In the dream, a beautiful woman led him through unknown landscapes until they came to a large cemetery. Many corpses lay on the ground, and in the center stood a large white tent covered with ornate decorations and surrounded by beautiful flowers. In the center of the tent, a brown woman sat on a large throne. She wore a white dress and her hair was ornamented with turquoise and gold. Many beautiful dakinis were gathered around her, speaking the languages of many different countries, and Tongjung Thuchen realized they had come from distant lands.

Leaving her throne, the brown dakini brought Tongjung Thuchen a skull full of blood and flesh and fed him from it. As she did so, she told him to accept the offerings as pure offerings, and that she and the other dakinis were going to give him an important initiation.

Then she said, "May you achieve enlightenment in the space of the Great Mother. I am Sippe Gyalmo, the holder of the Bön teaching, the Brown Queen of Existence. This initiation and teaching is the quintessential root *Mother Tantra*. I initiate you so that you can initiate and teach this to others." Tongjung Thuchen was led to a high throne. Sippe Gyalmo then gave him a ceremonial hat, an initiation robe, and ritual implements. She then surprised him by requesting that he give initiation to the gathered dakinis.

Tongjung Thuchen said, "Oh no, I can't give initiation. I don't know how to do this initiation. This is very embarrassing."

Sippe Gyalmo reassured him, "Don't worry. You are a great master. You have all the initiations from the thirty masters of Tibet and Zhang Zhung. You can give us initiation."

"I don't know how to sing the prayers during the initiation," Tongjung Thuchen objected.

Sippe Gyalmo said, "I'll help you and all the protectors will give you power. There is nothing to be afraid of. Please, do the initiation."

At that point, all of the meat and blood in the tent transformed into butter, sugar, and various foodstuffs, and into medicine and flowers. The dakinis tossed flowers on him. Suddenly he realized that he did know how to give the initiation for the *Mother Tantra* and he did so.

Afterwards all the dakinis thanked him. Sippe Gyalmo said, "In five years the dakinis from the eight major cemeteries will meet as will many masters. If you come, we will give you more teachings from the *Mother Tantra*." Then the dakinis all said goodbye to him, and he to them, and Sippe Gyalmo told him he was to leave. A red dakini wrote a *YAM* syllable on a scarf, representing the wind element, and waved it in the air, then asked him to touch the scarf with his right foot. The moment he did, he was back in his body and realized that he was sleeping.

He slept for a such a long time that people thought he was dead. When he finally woke, his master asked him why he had slept so long. He recounted the dream to his master, who told him that it was quite wonderful, but also cautioned him to keep it secret lest it become an obstacle. The master told Tongjung Thuchen that someday he would be a teacher and then gave him a blessing to empower his future teachings.

The following year, Tongjung Thuchen was in retreat when one evening he was visited by three dakinis. They had green scarves that they touched to his feet. As they did so, he lost consciousness briefly, and then woke in a dream.

He saw three caves facing East. A beautiful lake was in front of the caves. He walked into the central cave. Inside, it was wonderfully decorated with flowers. He met three masters, each dressed differently in esoteric initiation clothes. They were surrounded by lovely dakinis who played musical instruments, danced, made offerings, prayed, and performed other sacred activities.

The three masters gave him initiations to wake him to the natural state, to cause him to remember his past lives, and to enable him to teach the chöd practice successfully. The central master stood and said, "You have all the sacred teachings. You have received the initiations and we have blessed you to empower your ability to teach."

Then the master who sat to the right rose and said, "We initiate you into all the general teachings, the logical philosophies used to cut the ego, the use of the conceptual mind to liberate delusions, and into the chöd practices. We bless you so that you can teach these practices and give them continuity."

The master on the left then stood and said, "I'm going to give you the sacred tantric teaching that is at the heart of all the masters of Tibet and Zhang Zhung. We initiate you and bless you through these teachings so that you can help others."

All three masters were very important Bön masters who had lived around the end of the seventh century, over five hundred years before Tongjung Thuchen was born.

Some time later, after Tongjung Thuchen's master had passed away, Tongjung Thuchen returned to his master's little village where he did rituals and practices for the people there. On numerous occasions, during both short meditations and retreats, he was visited by various masters in visions. He experienced being able to see inside his own body, with the channels and energies appearing as clear crystal. Many times when he walked his feet did not touch the ground, and he could walk very, very fast, using the power of his prana.

Four more years passed. The brown dakini he had met in his dream, the manifestation of Sippe Gyalmo, had told him they would meet again after five years and the time had arrived. One day he took a nap in a cave and during sleep prayed to all the masters. When he awoke, he looked into an incredibly clear sky. A small breeze arose and two dakinis came to him, riding the wind, and told him that he was to accompany them.

He went with them to a gathering of dakinis, the same dakinis from many lands whom he had met in the dream five years earlier. He received transmissions and explanations of the chöd practices and the *Mother Tantra*. The dakinis predicted that in the future a time would arrive in which bodhisattvas and twelve blessed masters would appear and that during that time Tongjung Thuchen would teach. Each dakini made a promise to aid him in teaching. One said that she would act as a guardian of the teachings, another said that she would bless the teachings, the next said that she would protect the teachings from erroneous words and interpretations, and so on. Sippe Gyalmo also pledged to act as a protector of the teachings. In turn, each of the assembled dakinis told him what responsibilities she would undertake to aid the spread of the teachings, and they told him that the teachings would spread in the ten directions like the rays of the sun, to all the areas of the world. That prophecy was an important one that is encouraging for those who today learn these practices, because we know that they are going to spread out across the earth.

Tongjung Thuchen's dreams are good examples of dreams of clarity. He received accurate information in one dream regarding an important dream he would have in the future. He received teachings and initiations and was aided by dakinis and other masters. In the early part of his life, though he was accomplished, he did not know his full potential as a master until it was revealed to him in dream. Through the blessings he received in dream, he woke to different dimensions of consciousness and was reconnected to the part of himself that had learned and developed in past lives. He continued growing through his dreams, receiving teachings and meeting with masters and dakinis throughout his life.

So it can be with all of us. We will find, as practitioners, that a continuity develops in that part of our life we spend in dream. This is valuable in our spiritual journey, as dream becomes part of a specific process that reconnects us to our deeper selves, and matures our spiritual development.

4 Two Levels of Practice

One night, some years ago, I dreamed that a snake was in my mouth. I pulled it out and found that it was dead; it was quite unpleasant. An ambulance arrived at my house and the paramedics told me the snake was poisonous and that I was dying. I said okay, and they took me to the hospital.

I was afraid and told them I needed to see a statue of Tapihritsa, the Dzogchen master, before I died. The paramedics did not know who he was, but they agreed and told me I would have to wait to die, which relieved me. But then they surprised me by bringing the statue right away. My excuse for delaying death had not worked for very long. So I then told them there was no death; this was now my crutch. And the minute I said that, I awoke with a rapidly beating heart.

It was New Year's Eve and the next day I was to fly to Rome from Houston. Feeling uncomfortable after the dream, I thought that perhaps I should take it seriously and cancel my travel plans. I wanted my teacher's advice, so I went back to sleep and in a lucid dream traveled to Lopon in Nepal and told him of the disturbing dream.

At that time, Houston was having a lot of trouble with flooding. My teacher interpreted the dream to mean that I was representing Garuda, the mystic bird that has power over the Nagas, the snake-like water spirits. Lopon said that the dream meant that Garuda was conquering the water spirits that were the causes of the flooding. This interpretation made me feel much better; the next day I went to Rome as planned. This is an example of using lucid dream for something practical, for making decisions.

Perhaps this all sounds strange or unbelievable, but the real point is to develop the flexibility of the mind and to pierce the boundaries that constrict it. With greater flexibility, we can better accept what arises without being influenced by expectations and desires. Even while we are still limited by grasping and aversion, this kind of spiritual practice will benefit our daily lives.

If I am truly living in the realization that there is no death and no one to die, then I will not seek interpretation of a dream as I did in this case, when the dream left me feeling anxious. Our desire for interpretation of a dream is based on hope and fear; we want to know what to avoid and what to promote, we want to obtain understanding in order to change something. When you realize your true nature you do not seek meaning, for who would be doing the seeking? As you are then beyond hope and fear, the meaning of a dream becomes unimportant; you simply experience fully whatever manifests in the present moment. No dream, then, can cause anxiety.

Dream yoga spans the whole of our lives and applies to all the different dimensions of our experience. This can lead to a sense of a conflict between the highest philosophic view and some of the instructions. On the one hand, the view is boundless: the teachings that apply to non-duality, to non-conventional reality, declare that there is nothing to accomplish, that seeking is losing, that effort carries one away from one's true nature. But there are also practices and teachings that only make sense in terms of duality, in terms of hope and fear. Instruction is given on interpreting dreams, on pacifying local guardians, on accomplishing long-life practices, and the student is urged to practice with diligence and to guard the focus of the mind. It sounds like we are being told both that there is nothing to accomplish and that we need to work very hard.

Sometimes confusion on this point leads a practitioner into confusion regarding practice. The question arises: "If ultimate reality is empty of distinctions, and if liberation is to be found in the realization of this empty nature, then why should I do practices that are aimed at relative results?" The answer is very simple. Because we live in a dualistic, relative world, we do practices that are effective in this world. In samsaric existence, dichotomies and polarities have meaning; there is right and wrong, and better and worse ways to act and to think, based on the values of different religions, spiritual schools, philosophical systems, science, and culture. Respect the circumstances in which you are bound. When living in samsara, conventional practices apply and dream interpretation can be very helpful.

I needed the interpretation of the dream because I was afraid of death. But it is important for me to know that my need was based on fear, on dualism, and that when I abide in non-dual presence there is no fear and I need no interpretation. We use what is useful for the situation in which we find ourselves. When we live only in the nature of the mind, the state in which reality truly is void of distinctions, then we do not need to do relative practices. Then there is no need for the interpretation of dream because there is no need to redirect ourselves, there is no egoic self to redirect. We do not need to consult a dream about the future, because there is no hope or fear. We are completely present in whatever arises, without aversion or attraction. We do not need to look to the dream for meaning, because we are living in the truth.

In our conventional lives, we make choices and can change things; that is why we study the teachings, why we practice. As we understand more and become more skilled in our lives, we become more flexible. We begin to really understand the things that we are taught: what lucidity is, what is illusory about our experiences, how suffering comes about, what our true nature is. Once we start to see how what we do is a cause of more suffering, we can then choose to do something different. We grow weary of constricted identities and the repetitive inclinations that lead to so much unnecessary suffering. We let go of negative emotional states, train ourselves to overcome distraction, and abide in pure presence.

It is the same with dreaming. There is a progression in the practice. As the practice is developed, it is discovered that there is another way to dream. Then we move toward the unconventional dream practices in which the story and its interpretations are not important. We work more on the causes of dreams than the dreams themselves.

There is no reason not to use dream yoga to attain worldly goals. Some of the practices address relative concerns and lead to the use of dreaming for purposes such as health, divination, guidance, cleansing unhealthy karmic and psychological tendencies, healing, and so on. The path is practical and suited for all. But, while the use of dream yoga to benefit us in the relative world is good, it is a provisional use of dream. Ultimately we want to use dream to liberate ourselves from all relative conditions, not simply to improve them.

PART THREE

The Practice of Dream Yoga

1 Vision, Action, Dream, Death

The *Mother Tantra* says that if one is not aware in vision, it is unlikely that one will be aware in behavior. If one is not aware in behavior, one is unlikely to be aware in dream. And if one is not aware in dream, then one is unlikely to be aware in the bardo after death.

What does this mean? "Vision" in this context does not mean simply visual phenomena, but rather the totality of experience. It includes every perception, sensation, and mental and emotional event, as well as everything that seems external to us. Vision is what we "see" as experience; it is our experience. Being unaware in vision means being unable to see the truth of what arises in experience and instead being deluded by the misunderstandings of the dualistic mind, mistaking the projections and fantasies of that mind for reality.

When we lack awareness of the true situation in which we exist, it is difficult to respond skillfully to what we encounter in both external and internal life. Instead, we react according to the karmic habits of grasping and aversion, driven this way and that by unhappiness and illusory hopes. Taking action based on these confusions is what is meant by lack of awareness in behavior. The result of such action is the reinforcement of attachment, hatred, and ignorance and the creation of further negative karmic traces.

Dreams arise from the same karmic traces that govern our waking experiences. If we are too distracted to penetrate the fantasies and delusions of the moving mind during the day, we will most likely be bound by the same limitations in dream. This is "not being aware in dream." The dream phenomena we encounter will evoke in us the same emotions and dualistic reactions in which we are lost when awake, and it will be difficult to develop lucidity or engage in the further practices.

We enter the bardo, the intermediate state after death, just as we enter dream after falling asleep. If our experience of dream lacks clarity and is of confused emotional states and habitual reactivity, we will have trained ourselves to experience the processes of death in the same way. We will be driven into further karmic bondage by reacting dualistically to the visions in the intermediate state, and our future rebirth will be determined by whatever karmic tendencies we have cultivated in life. This is "lacking awareness in the bardo."

Conversely, when we continually bring awareness to the immediate moment of experience, this capacity will soon be found in dream. As we cultivate presence in dream, we prepare ourselves for death. Dream practice is correlated to this progression.

In order to progress we must develop some stability in the mind so that we can maintain greater awareness in experience, in "vision," and develop the capacity for skillful responsiveness. Therefore, the first practice is calm abiding (zhiné), in which the mind is trained to be still, focused, and alert.

As we bring greater awareness to experience, we can overcome the habits of reaction based on the delusions of the conventional mind. The four foundational practices further this flexibility by training the mind to use every object of waking experience as a cause for increased lucidity and presence. As we loosen the grip of karmic reactivity, we are able to choose to act positively. This is bringing awareness to behavior.

The awareness we have stabilized during waking experience and manifested in our behaviors naturally begins to arise in the dream. The primary practices use the understanding of the prana, chakras, and mind to support this strengthening of awareness in the dream. They are done before falling asleep and in three waking periods during the night. Once lucidity is developed there are further practices engaged during the dream itself in order to develop flexibility of mind, to break the limitations and misunderstandings that bind us to samsara.

Just as the lucidity and presence cultivated in waking life is carried into the dream, the lucidity and presence cultivated in dream is carried into death. If one fully accomplishes dream yoga, one is prepared to enter the intermediate state after death with the correct view and the stability in non-dual presence needed to attain liberation.

This is the sequence: awareness in the first moment of experience, in response, in dream, and then in death. One cannot just start at the end. You can determine for yourself how mature your practice is: as you encounter the phenomena of experience, examine your feelings and your reactions to the feelings. Are you controlled by your interactions with the objects of experience or do you control your reactions to them? Are you thrown into emotional reactions by your attractions and aversions, or can you remain in steady presence in diverse situations? If the former, practice will cultivate the presence needed to free you of karmic conditioning and reactivity. If the latter, you will increasingly develop stability in awareness and your dreams will change in extraordinary ways.

2 Calm Abiding: Zhiné

A successful dream yogi must be stable enough in presence to avoid being swept away by the winds of karmic emotions and lost in the dream. As the mind steadies, dreams become longer, less fragmented, and more easily remembered, and lucidity is developed. Waking life is equally enhanced as we find that we are increasingly protected from being carried away by the habitual emotional reactions that draw us into distraction and unhappiness, and can instead develop the positive traits that lead to happiness and that support us in the spiritual journey.

All yogic and spiritual disciplines include some form of practice that develops concentration and quiets the mind. In the Tibetan tradition this practice is called calm abiding (zhiné). We recognize three stages in the development of stability: forceful zhiné, natural zhiné, and ultimate zhiné. Zhiné begins with mental fixation on an object and, when concentration is strong enough, moves on to fixation without an object.

Begin the practice by sitting in the five-pointed meditation posture: the legs crossed, the hands folded in the lap in meditation position with palms up and placed one on top of the other, the spine straight but not rigid, the head tilted down slightly to straighten the neck, and the eyes open. The eyes should be relaxed, not too wide open and not too closed. The object of concentration should be placed so that the eyes can look straight ahead, neither up nor down. During the practice try not to move, not even to swallow or blink, while keeping the mind one-pointedly on the object. Even if tears should stream down your face, do not move. Let the breathing be natural.

Generally, for practice with an object, we use the Tibetan letter *A* as the object of concentration. This letter has many symbolic meanings but here is used simply as a support for the development of focus. Other objects may also be used—the letter *A* of the English alphabet, an image, the sound of a mantra, the breath—almost anything. However, it is good to use something connected to the sacred, as it serves to inspire you. Also, try to use the same object each time you practice, rather than switching between objects, because the continuity acts as a support of the practice. It is also somewhat preferable to focus on a

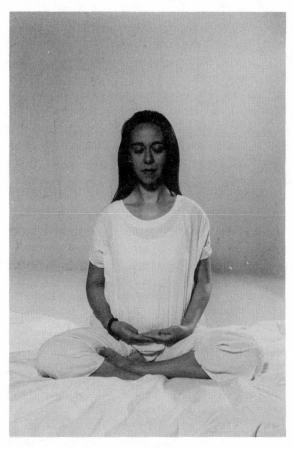

Meditation Posture

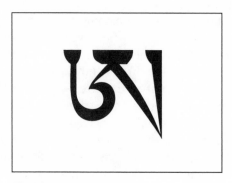

The Tibetan A

physical object that is outside the body, as the purpose is to develop stability during the perception of external objects and, eventually, of the objects in dream.

If you wish to use the Tibetan *A* you can write it on a piece of paper about an inch square. Traditionally, the letter is white and is enclosed in five concentric colored circles: the center circle that is the direct background for the *A* is indigo; around it is a blue circle, then green, red, yellow, and white ones. Tape the paper to a stick that is just long enough to support the paper at eye level when you sit for practice, and make a base that holds it upright. Place it so that the *A* is about a foot and a half in front of your eyes.

Many signs of progress can arise during the practice. As concentration strengthens and the periods of practice are extended, strange sensations arise in the body and many strange visual phenomena appear. You may find your mind doing strange things, too! That is all right. These experiences are a natural part of the development of concentration; they arise as the mind settles, so be neither disturbed by nor excited about them.

FORCEFUL ZHINÉ

The first stage of practice is called "forceful" because it requires effort. The mind is easily and quickly distracted, and it may seem impossible to remain focused on the object for even a minute. In the beginning, it is helpful to practice in numerous short sessions alternating with breaks. Do not let the mind wander during the break, but instead recite a mantra, or work with visualization, or work with another practice you may know, such as the development of compassion. After the break, return to the fixation practice. If you are ready to practice but do not have the particular object you have been using, visualize a ball of light on your forehead and center yourself there. The practice should be done once or twice a day, and can be done more frequently if you have the time. Developing concentration is like strengthening the muscles of the body: exercise must be done regularly and frequently. To become stronger keep pushing against your limits.

Keep the mind on the object. Do not follow the thoughts of the past or the future. Do not allow the attention to be carried away by fantasy, sound, physical sensation, or any other distraction. Just remain in the sensuality of the present moment, and with your whole strength and clarity focus the mind through the eye, on the object. Do not lose the awareness of the object even for a second. Breathe gently, and then more gently, until the sense of breathing is lost. Slowly allow yourself to enter more deeply into quiet and calm. Make certain that the body is kept relaxed; do not tense up in concentration. Neither should you allow yourself to fall into a stupor, a dullness, or a trance.

Do not think about the object, just let it be in awareness. This is an important distinction to make. Thinking about the object is not the kind of concentration we are developing. The point is just to keep the mind placed on the object, on the sense perception of the object, to undistractedly remain aware of the presence of the object. When the mind does get distracted—and it often will in the beginning—gently bring it back to the object and leave it there.

NATURAL ZHINÉ

As stability is developed, the second stage of practice is entered: natural zhiné. In the first stage, concentration is developed by continually directing the attention to the object and developing control over the unruly mind. In the second stage, the mind is absorbed in contemplation of the object and there is no longer the need for force to hold it still. A relaxed and pleasant tranquility is established, in which the mind is quiet and thoughts arise without distracting the mind from the object. The elements of the body become harmonized and the prana moves evenly and gently throughout the body. This is an appropriate time to move to fixation without an object.

Abandoning the physical object, simply fix the focus on space. It is helpful to gaze into expansive space, like the sky, but the practice can be done even in a small room by fixing on the space between your body and the wall. Remain steady and calm. Leave the body relaxed.

Rather than focusing on an imagined point in space, allow the mind, while remaining in strong presence, to be diffuse. We call this "dissolving the mind" in space, or "merging the mind with space." It will lead to stable tranquility and the third stage of zhiné practice.

ULTIMATE ZHINÉ

Whereas in the second stage there is still some heaviness involved in the absorption in the object, the third stage is characterized by a mind that is tranquil but light, relaxed, and pliable. Thoughts arise and dissolve spontaneously and without effort. The mind is integrated fully with its own movement.

In the Dzogchen tradition, this is traditionally when the master introduces the student to the natural state of mind. Because the student has developed zhiné, the master can point to what the student has already experienced rather than describing a new state that must be attained. The explanation, which is known as the "pointing out" instruction, is meant to lead the student to recognize what is already there, to discriminate the moving mind in thought and concept from the nature of mind, which is pure, non-dual awareness. This is the ultimate stage of zhiné practice, abiding in non-dual presence, rigpa itself.

OBSTACLES

In developing the zhiné practice, there are three obstacles that must be overcome: agitation, drowsiness, and laxity.

Agitation

Agitation causes the mind to jump restlessly from one thought to another and makes concentration difficult. To prevent this, calm yourself before the practice session by avoiding too much physical or mental activity. Slow stretches may help to relax the body and quiet the mind. Once you are sitting, take a few deep, slow breaths. Make it a practice to focus the mind immediately when you start the practice to avoid developing the habit of mentally wandering while sitting in meditation posture.

Drowsiness

The second obstacle is drowsiness or sleepiness, which moves into the mind like a fog, a heaviness and torpor that blunts awareness. When it does this, try to strengthen the mind's focus on the object in order to penetrate the drowsiness. You may find that drowsiness is actually a kind of movement of the mind that you can stop with strong concentration. If this does not work, take a break, stretch, and perhaps do some practice while standing.

Laxity

The third obstacle is laxity. When encountering this obstacle you may feel that your mind is calm, but in a passive, weak mental state in which the concentration has no strength. It is important to recognize this state for what it is. It can be a pleasant and relaxed experience and, if mistaken for correct meditation, may cause the practitioner to spend years mistakenly cultivating it, with no discernable change in the quality of consciousness. If your focus loses strength and your practice becomes lax, straighten your posture and wake up your mind. Reinforce the attention and guard the stability of presence. Regard the practice as something precious, which it is, and as something that will lead to the attainment of the highest realization, which it will. Strengthen the intention and automatically the wakefulness of the mind is strengthened.

Zhiné practice should be done every day until the mind is quiet and stable. It is not only a preliminary practice, but is helpful at any point in the practitioner's life; even very advanced yogis practice zhiné. The stability of mind developed through zhiné is the foundation of dream yoga and all other meditation practices. Once we have achieved a strong and reliable steadiness in calm presence, we can develop this steadiness in all aspects of life. When stable, this presence can always be found, and we will not be carried away by thoughts and emotions. Then, even though karmic traces continue to produce dream images after falling asleep, we remain in awareness. This opens the door to the further practices of both dream and sleep yogas.

3   The Four Foundational Practices

There are four main foundational practices in dream yoga. Although they are traditionally called the Four Preparations, this does not mean that they are of lesser importance and are to followed by the "real" practice. They are preparatory in the sense that they are the foundations upon which success in the primary practice depends.

Dream yoga is rooted in the way the mind is used during waking life, and it is this that the foundational practices address. How the mind is used determines the kinds of dreams that arise in sleep as well as the quality of waking life. Change the way you relate to the objects and people of waking life and you change the experience of dream. After all, the "you" that lives the dream of waking life is the same "you" that lives the dream of sleeping life. If you spend the day spaced out and caught up in the elaborations of the conceptual mind, you are likely to do the same in dream. And if you are more present when awake, you will also find that presence in dream.

ONE: CHANGING THE KARMIC TRACES

A version of the first foundational practice is rather well known in the West, because dream researchers and others interested in dream have found that it helps to generate lucid dreaming. It is as follows: throughout the day, practice the recognition of the dream-like nature of life until the same recognition begins to manifest in dream.

Upon waking in the morning, think to yourself, "I am awake in a dream." When you enter the kitchen, recognize it as a dream kitchen.

Pour dream milk into dream coffee. "It's all a dream," you think to yourself, "this is a dream." Remind yourself of this constantly throughout the day.

The emphasis should actually be on you, the dreamer, more than on the objects of your experience. Keep reminding yourself that you are dreaming up your experiences: the anger you feel, the happiness, the fatigue, the anxiety—it is all part of the dream. The oak tree you appreciate, the car you drive, the person to whom you are talking, are all part of the dream. In this way a new tendency is created in the mind, that of looking at experience as insubstantial, transient, and intimately related to the mind's projections. As phenomena are seen to be fleeting and essenceless, grasping decreases. Every sensory encounter and mental event becomes a reminder of the dream-like nature of experience. Eventually this understanding will arise in dream and lead to the recognition of the dream state and the development of lucidity.

There are two ways to understand the declaration that everything is a dream. The first is to look upon it as a method to change the karmic traces. Doing this practice, like all practices, changes the way one engages the world. By changing habitual and largely unconscious reactions to phenomena, the qualities of life and dream change. When we think of an experience as "only a dream" it is less "real" to us. It loses power over us—power that it only had because we gave it power—and can no longer disturb us and drive us into negative emotional states. Instead, we begin to encounter all experience with greater calm and increased clarity, and even with greater appreciation. In this sense, the practice works psychologically by altering the meaning that we project onto what is beyond conceptual meaning. As we view experience differently, we change our reaction to it, which changes the karmic remnants of actions, and the root of dreaming changes.

The second way of understanding the practice is to realize that waking life is actually the same as dream, that the entirety of normal experience is made up of the mind's projections, that all meaning is imputed, and that whatever we experience is due to the influence of karma. Here we are talking about the subtle and pervasive work of karma, the endless cycle of cause and effect that creates the present from the traces of the past, which it does through the continual conditioning that results from every action. This is one way of articulating the realization that all phenomena are empty and that the apparent self-nature of beings and objects is illusory. There is not an actual "thing" anywhere in waking life—just as in a dream—but only transient, essenceless appearances, arising and self-liberating in the empty, luminous base of existence. Fully realizing the truth of the statement, "This is a dream," we are freed of the habits of erroneous conception and therefore freed from the diminished life of samsara in which fantasy is mistaken for reality. We are necessarily present when this realization comes, as it is then true that there is no place else to be. And there is no stronger method of bringing consistent lucidity to dream than by abiding continuously in lucid presence during the day.

As stated above, an important part of this practice is to experience yourself as a dream. Imagine yourself as an illusion, as a dream figure, with a body that lacks solidity. Imagine your personality and various identities as projections of mind. Maintain presence, the same lucidity you are trying to cultivate in dream, while sensing yourself as insubstantial and transient, made only of light. This creates a very different relationship with yourself that is comfortable, flexible, and expansive.

In doing these practices, it is not enough to simply repeat again and again that you are in a dream. The truth of the statement must be felt and experienced beyond the words. Use the imagination, senses, and awareness in fully integrating the practice with felt experience. When you do the practice properly, each time you think that you are in a dream, presence becomes stronger and experience more vivid. If there is not this kind of immediate qualitative change, make certain that the practice has not become only the mechanical repetition of a phrase, which is of little benefit. There is no magic in just thinking a formula; the words should be used to remind yourself to bring greater awareness and calm to the moment. When practicing the recognition, "wake" yourself—by increasing clarity and presence—again and again until just remembering the thought, "This is a dream," brings a simultaneous strengthening and brightening of awareness

This is the first preparation, to see all life as a dream. It is to be applied in the moment of perception and before a reaction arises. It is a potent practice in itself and greatly affects the practitioner. Remain in this awareness and you will experience lucidity both while awake and during dream.

There is one warning regarding this practice: it is important to take care of responsibilities and to respect the logic and limitations of conventional life. When you tell yourself that your waking life is a dream, this is true, but if you leap from a building you will still fall, not fly.

If you do not go to work, bills will go unpaid. Plunge your hand in a fire and you will be burned. It is important to remain grounded in the realities of the relative world, because as long as there is a "you" and "me," there is a relative world in which we live, other sentient beings who are suffering, and consequences from the decisions we make.

TWO: REMOVING GRASPING AND AVERSION

The second foundational practice works to further decrease grasping and aversion. Whereas the first preparation is applied in the moment of encountering phenomena and before a reaction occurs, the second practice is engaged after a reaction has arisen. Essentially they are the same practice, distinguished only by the situation in which the practice is applied and by the object of attention. The first practice directs lucid awareness and the recognition of phenomena as a dream toward everything that is encountered: sense objects, internal events, one's own body, and so forth. The second preparation specifically directs the same lucid awareness to emotionally shaded reactions that occur in response to the elements of experience.

Ideally the practice should be applied as soon as any grasping or aversion arises in response to an object or situation. The grasping mind may manifest its reaction as desire, anger, jealousy, pride, envy, grief, despair, joy, anxiety, depression, fear, boredom, or any other emotional reaction.

When a reaction arises, remind yourself that you, the object, and your reaction to the object are all dream. Think to yourself, "This anger is a dream. This desire is a dream. This indignation, grief, exuberance, is a dream." The truth in this statement becomes clear when you pay attention to the inner processes that produce emotional states: you literally dream them up through a complex interaction of thoughts, images, bodily states, and sensations. Emotional reactivity does not originate "out there" in objects. It arises, is experienced, and ceases in you.

There is an infinite variety of stimuli to which you may react: attraction may arise at the sight of a beautiful man or woman, anger at a driver that cuts in front of you, disgust or sorrow at a ruined environment, anxiety and worry about a situation or person, and so on. Every situation and reaction should be recognized as a dream. Do not just slap the sentence onto a piece of your experience; try to actually feel the dream-like quality of your inner life. When this assertion is actually felt, not just thought, the relationship to the situation changes, and the tight, emotional grip on phenomena relaxes. The situation becomes clearer and more spacious, and grasping and aversion are directly recognized as the uncomfortable constrictions that they truly are. This is a powerful antidote to the state of near possession and obsession that negative emotional states create. Direct and certain experience of using this practice to untie the knot of negative emotion is the beginning of the real practice of lucidity and flexibility that leads to consequent freedom. With consistent practice, even strong states of anger, depression, and other states of unhappiness can be released. When they are, they dissolve.

The teachings generally refer to this particular practice as a method to give up attachments. There are healthy and unhealthy ways to give these up. It does one little good to suppress desires; they are then transformed into internal turmoil or external condemnations and intolerance. And it also works against spiritual development to attempt to flee from pain through distraction or by tightening the body in order to choke off experience. It can be healthy to give up worldly life and become a monk or a nun or it can be an unhealthy attempt to escape difficult experiences through suppression and avoidance.

Dream yoga cuts attachment by reorganizing the perception and understanding of the object or situation, by altering the view and thus allowing the practitioner to see through the illusory appearance of an object to its radiant, light-like reality. As the practice progresses, objects and situations are not only experienced with greater clarity and vividness but are also recognized as ephemeral, insubstantial, and fleeting. This levels the relative importance of phenomena and diminishes the grasping and aversion based on preference.

THREE: STRENGTHENING INTENTION

The third preparation involves reviewing the day before going to sleep, and strengthening the intention to practice during the night. As you prepare for sleep, allow the memories of the day to arise. Whatever comes to mind recognize as a dream. The memories most likely to arise are of those experiences strong enough to affect the coming dreams. During this review, attempt to experience the memories that arise as memories of dreams. Memory is actually very similar to dream. Again, this is not about automatic labeling, a ritual of repeating "It was a dream," over and over. Try to truly comprehend the dream-like nature of your experience, the projections that sustain it, and feel the difference of relating to experience as a dream.

Then develop the strong determination to recognize the dreams of the night for what they are. Make the strongest intention possible to know directly and vividly, while dreaming, that you are dreaming. The intention is like an arrow that awareness can follow during the night, an arrow directed at lucidity in dream. The Tibetan phrase we use for generating intention translates as "sending a wish." We should have that sense here, that we are making prayers and intentions and sending them to our teachers and to the buddhas and deities, promising to try to remain in awareness and asking for their help. There are other practices that can be done before falling asleep, but this one is available to all.

FOUR: CULTIVATING MEMORY AND JOYFUL EFFORT

The fourth foundational practice is engaged upon awaking in the morning. It further cultivates strong intention and also strengthens the capacity to remember the events of the night.

Begin by reviewing the night. The Tibetan term for this preparation is literally "remembering." Did you dream? Were you aware that you were in a dream? If you dreamt but did not attain lucidity, you should reflect, "I dreamt but did not recognize the dream as a dream. But it was a dream." Resolve that next time you enter a dream you will become aware of its true nature while still in the dream.

If you find it difficult to remember dreams, it can be helpful, throughout the day and particularly before sleep, to generate a strong intention to remember dreams. You can also record dreams in a notepad or with a tape recorder, as this will reinforce the habit of treating your dreams as something valuable. The very act of preparing the notebook or recorder at night serves to support the intention to recall the dream upon waking. It is not difficult for anyone to remember dreams once the intention to do so is generated and sustained, even over just a few days.

If you did have a lucid dream, feel joy at the accomplishment. Develop happiness relative to the practice and resolve to continue to develop the lucidity the following night. Keep building intention, using both successes and failures as occasions to develop ever stronger intent to accomplish the practice. And know that even your intention is a dream.

Finally, during the morning period, generate a strong intention to remain consistent in the practice throughout the day. And pray with your full heart for success; prayer is like a magical power that we all have and forget to use.

This practice merges into the first foundational practice, recognizing all experience as a dream. In this fashion the practice becomes uninterrupted around the wheel of day and night.

CONSISTENCY

The importance of the four preparations to the later stages of dream yoga cannot be overstated. They are much more powerful than they may appear to be. Furthermore, they are practices anyone can do. They are more psychologically oriented than many practices and will present no difficulty for the practitioner. Simply doing a practice before going to bed may be ineffective, but with consistent practice of the preparations during the day it becomes much easier to attain lucidity in dream and to then go on to the further practices. Using these practices makes everything that happens a cause for the return to presence, and this will bring great benefit to daily life as well as lead to success in dream yoga.

If you do not have immediate results, even if you must practice for a long time before achieving lucidity in dream, there is no need to be discouraged. Do not think that it is useless and that you cannot accomplish the practice. Think about the differences in how you thought and acted when you were ten years old, relative to now—there is constant change. Do not allow yourself to get stuck, believing that whatever limits you have in your practice today will continue in the future. Knowing that nothing remains the same, you need not believe that the way things manifest now are the way they must continue.

Experiencing the vivid, luminous, dream-like qualities of life allows your experience to grow more spacious, lighter, and clearer. When lucidity is developed in dream and in waking, there is much greater freedom to shape life positively, and to finally give up preferences and dualisms altogether and remain in non-dual presence.

4 Preparation for the Night

The average person, not knowing the principles of meditation, carries the stress, emotions, thoughts, and confusions of the day into the night. For such a person there is no particular practice or time set aside for processing the day or calming down before entering sleep. Instead, sleep comes in the midst of distraction, and negativities are held in the mind throughout the night. When dream arises from those negativities, there is no stability in presence and the individual is carried away by the images and confusions of the dream world. The body remains tense with anxiety, or heavy with sadness, and the prana in the body is rough and uneven as the mind darts here and there. Sleep is disturbed, dreams are stressful or merely a pleasant escape, and the sleeper wakes tired and unrested in the morning, often continuing through the day in a negative state.

Even for one who does not practice dream or sleep yogas, it is beneficial to prepare for sleep, to take it seriously. Purifying the mind as much as possible before sleep, just as before meditating, generates more presence and positive qualities. Rather than carrying negative emotions into the night, use whatever skills you have to free yourself from such emotions. If you know how to allow the emotion to self-liberate, to dissolve into emptiness, do so. If you know how to transform it or provide the antidote, then use that knowledge. Try to connect with the lama, yidam*, and dakini; pray to the Buddhas and deities; generate compassion. Do what you can to rid yourself of tension in the body and negative attitudes in the mind. Free of disturbance, with a light and easy mind, you will experience a sleep that is more restful and healing. Even if there is an inability to do the rest of the practices, this practice is something positive that everyone can incorporate into daily life.

Below are some general preparations for the night, but do not limit yourself to these. The important point is to be aware of what you are doing with your mind and how it is affecting you, and to use your knowledge to calm yourself, become present, and open up the possibilities of the night.

NINE PURIFICATIONS BREATHING

Perhaps you have noticed how much tension is carried in the body and how the tension affects breathing. When someone with whom we are having difficulties walks into the room, the body tightens and the breath becomes shorter and sharper. When we are frightened, the breath comes quick and shallow. In sadness, the breathing is often deep and punctuated by sighs. And if someone we genuinely like and care for enters the room, the body relaxes and the breath opens and eases.

Rather than waiting for experience to alter the breath, we can deliberately alter the breath to change our experience. The nine breaths of purification is a short practice to clear and purify the channels and relax the mind and body. The drawings of the channels can be found on page 47.

Sit in a cross-legged meditation posture. Place your hands palm-up in your lap, with the left hand resting on the right. Bend your head just a little to straighten the neck.

Visualize the three channels of energy in your body. The central channel is blue and rises straight through the center of the body; it is the size of a cane, and widens slightly from the heart to its opening at the crown of the head. The side channels are the diameter of pencils and join the central channel at its base, about four inches below the navel. They rise straight through the body to either side of the central channel, curve around under the skull, pass down behind the eyes, and open at the nostrils. In women the right channel is red and the left is white. In men the right channel is white and the left is red.

First Three Breaths

Men: Raise the right hand with the thumb pressing the base of the ring finger. Closing the right nostril with the ring finger, inhale green light through the left nostril. Then, closing the left nostril with the right ring finger, exhale completely through the right nostril. Repeat this for three inhalations and exhalations.

Women: Raise the left hand with the thumb pressing the base of the ring finger. Closing the left nostril with the ring finger, inhale green light through the right nostril. Then, closing the right nostril with the ring finger, exhale completely through the left nostril. Repeat this for three inhalations and exhalations.

With each exhalation, imagine all obstacles linked with male potencies expelled from the white channel in the form of light-blue air. These include illnesses associated with the winds (pranas) as well as obstacles and obscurations connected with the past.

Second Three Breaths

Men and Women: Change hands and nostrils and repeat for three inhalations and exhalations. With each exhalation, imagine all obstacles linked with female potencies expelled from the red channel in the form of light-pink air. These include illnesses associated with bile as well as obstacles and obscurations associated with the future.

Third Three Breaths

Men and Women: Place the left hand on top of the right in the lap, palms up. Inhale green healing light into both nostrils. Visualize it moving down the side channels to the juncture with the main channel, four finger widths below the navel. With the exhalation, visualize the energy rising up the central channel and out the top of the head. Complete three inhalations and exhalations. With each exhalation, imagine all potencies for illnesses associated with hostile spirits expelled from the top of the head in the form of black smoke. These include illnesses associated with phlegm as well as obstacles and obscurations associated with the present.

GURU YOGA

Guru yoga is an essential practice in all schools of Tibetan Buddhism and Bön. This is true in sutra, tantra, and Dzogchen. It develops the heart connection with the master. By continually strengthening our devotion, we come to the place of pure devotion in ourselves, which is the unshakeable, powerful base of the practice. The essence of guru yoga is to merge the practitioner's mind with the mind of the master.

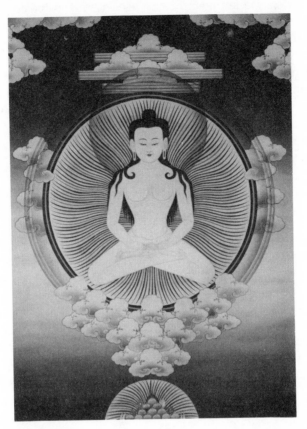

Tapihritsa

What is the true master? It is the formless, fundamental nature of mind, the primordial awareness of the base of everything, but because we exist in dualism, it is helpful for us to visualize this in a form. Doing so makes skillful use of the dualisms of the conceptual mind, to further strengthen devotion and help us stay directed toward practice and the generation of positive qualities.

In the Bön tradition, we often visualize either Tapihritsa* as the master, or the Buddha Shenla Odker*, who represents the union of all the masters. If you are already a practitioner, you may have another deity to visualize, like Guru Rinpoche or a yidam or dakini. While it is important to work with a lineage with which you have a connection, you should understand that the master you visualize is the embodiment of all the masters with whom you are connected, all the teachers with whom you have studied, all the deities to whom you have commitments. The master in guru yoga is not just one individual, but the essence of enlightenment, the primordial awareness that is your true nature.

The master is also the teacher from whom you receive the teachings. In the Tibetan tradition, we say the master is more important than the Buddha. Why? Because the master is the immediate messenger of the teachings, the one who brings the Buddha's wisdom to the student. Without the master we could not find our way to the Buddha. So we should feel as much devotion to the master as we would to the Buddha if the Buddha suddenly appeared in front of us.

Guru yoga is not just about generating some feeling toward a visualized image. It is done to find the fundamental mind in yourself that is the same as the fundamental mind of all your teachers, and of all the Buddhas and realized beings that have ever lived. When you merge with the guru, you merge with your pristine true nature, which is the real guide and master. But this should not be an abstract practice. When you do guru yoga, try to feel such intense devotion that the hair stands up on your neck, tears start down your face, and your heart opens and fills with great love. Let yourself merge in union with the guru's mind, which is your enlightened Buddha-nature. This is the way to practice guru yoga.

The Practice

After the nine breaths, still seated in meditation posture, visualize the master above and in front of you. This should not be a flat, two dimensional picture—let a real being exist there, in three dimensions, made of light, pure, and with a strong presence that affects the feeling in your body, your energy, and your mind. Generate strong devotion and reflect on the great gift of the teachings and the tremendous good fortune you enjoy in having made a connection to them. Offer a sincere prayer, asking that your negativities and obscurations be removed, that your positive qualities develop, and that you accomplish dream yoga.

Then imagine receiving blessings from the master in the form of three colored lights that stream from his or her three wisdom doors—of body, speech, and mind—into yours. The lights should be transmitted in the following sequence: White light streams from the master's brow chakra into yours, purifying and relaxing your entire body and physical dimension. Then red light streams from the master's throat chakra into yours, purifying and relaxing your energetic dimension. Finally, blue light streams from the master's heart chakra into yours, purifying and relaxing your mind.

When the lights enter your body, feel them. Let your body, energy, and mind relax, suffused in wisdom light. Use your imagination to make the blessing real in your full experience, in your body and energy as well as in the images in your mind.

After receiving the blessing, imagine the master dissolving into light that enters your heart and resides there as your innermost essence. Imagine that you dissolve into that light, and remain in pure awareness, rigpa.

There are more elaborate instructions for guru yoga that can involve prostrations, offerings, gestures, mantras, and more complicated visualizations, but the essence of the practice is mingling your mind with the mind of the master, which is pure, non-dual awareness. Guru yoga can be done any time during the day; the more often the better. Many masters say that of all the practices it is guru yoga that is the most important. It confers the blessings of the lineage and can open and soften the heart and quiet the unruly mind. To completely accomplish guru yoga is to accomplish the path.

PROTECTION

Going to sleep is a little like dying, a journey taken alone into the unknown. Ordinarily we are not troubled about sleep because we are familiar with it, but think about what it entails. We completely lose ourselves in a void for some period of time, until we arise again in a dream. When we do so, we may have a different identity and a different body. We may be in a strange place, with people we do not know, involved in baffling activities that may seem quite risky.

Just trying to sleep in an unfamiliar place may occasion anxiety. The place may be perfectly secure and comfortable, but we do not sleep as well as we do at home in familiar surroundings. Maybe the energy of the place feels wrong. Or maybe it is only our own insecurity that disturbs us, and even in familiar places we may feel anxious while waiting for sleep to come, or be frightened by what we dream. When we fall asleep with anxiety, our dreams are mingled with fear and tension, sleep is less restful, and the practice harder to do. So it is a good idea to create a sense of protection before we sleep and to turn our sleeping area into a sacred space.

This is done by imagining protective dakinis all around the sleeping area. Visualize the dakinis as beautiful goddesses, enlightened female beings who are loving, green in color, and powerfully protective. They remain near as you fall asleep and throughout the night, like mothers watching over their child, or guardians surrounding a king or queen. Imagine them everywhere, guarding the doors and the windows, sitting next to you on the bed, walking in the garden or the yard, and so on, until you feel completely protected.

Again, this practice is more than just trying to visualize something: see the dakinis with your mind but also use your imagination to feel their presence. Creating a protective, sacred environment in this way is calming and relaxing and promotes restful sleep. This is how the mystic lives: seeing the magic, changing the environment with the mind, and allowing actions, even actions of the imagination, to have significance.

You can enhance the sense of peace in your sleeping environment by keeping objects of a sacred nature in the bedroom: peaceful, loving images, sacred and religious symbols, and other objects that direct your mind toward the path.

The *Mother Tantra* tells us that as we prepare for sleep we should maintain awareness of the causes of dream, the object to focus upon, the protectors, and of ourselves. Hold these together in awareness, not as many things, but as a single environment, and this will have a great effect in dream and sleep.

5   The Main Practice

In order to fully develop dream yoga, there are four tasks that need to be accomplished in sequence: 1) bringing awareness into the central channel, 2) cultivating clear vision and experience, 3) developing power and strength so that we will not become lost, and 4) developing our wrathful aspect in order to overcome fear. These tasks correspond to the four qualities of dreams—peaceful, joyful, powerful, and wrathful—and to the four sections of the practice.

BRINGING AWARENESS INTO THE CENTRAL CHANNEL

After working with the preliminary practices during the day, and after doing the practices prior to sleep—purification breathing, guru yoga, generation of compassion and love, visualization of the protector dakinis, and forming of intention for the night—the first of the main practices is engaged.

Lie in the lion posture: Men lie on their right side, women on their left. Bend the knees enough to make the body stable, rest the top arm along the side, and place the lower hand under the cheek. You may benefit from experimenting with using a slightly higher pillow, being careful of your neck, in order to keep the sleep lighter. Gentle the breath and relax the body. Allow the breath to be full and very quiet so that neither the inhalation nor the exhalation can be heard.

Visualize a beautiful red lotus with four petals in the throat chakra. The throat chakra is at the base of the throat, closer to where the neck meets the shoulders than to the head. In the center of the four petals, facing forward, is an upright, luminous Tibetan *A*, clear and translucent, like crystal made of pure light. Just as a crystal laid on red cloth reflects the color and appears red, so does the *A* pick up the red of the petals and appear red. On each of the four petals is a syllable: *RA* to the front, *LA* to your left, *SHA* to the back, and *SA* to the right. As sleep comes, maintain a light, relaxed focus on the *A*.

This part of the practice is meant to bring the mind and prana into the central channel. The quality is peaceful, and as we merge with the deep red *A* we find peace within ourselves. The teaching says that focusing on this chakra produces gentle dreams. The example given is of a dream in which a dakini gently invites the dreamer to accompany

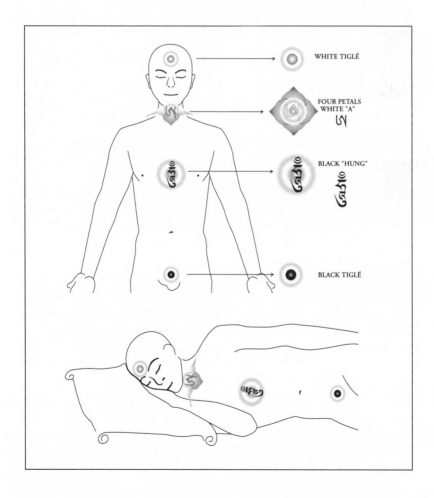

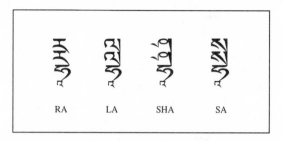

her. She helps the dreamer onto a mystical bird (garuda) or a lion and leads him or her to a pure land, a beautiful, sacred place. But the dream need not be this specific. It may just involve a walk in a beautiful garden or in the mountains, guided by other people. The quality of dreams generated has less to do with particular images and more to do, at this point, with the feeling of peace.

INCREASING CLARITY

After sleeping for approximately two hours, wake and engage in the second part of the practice. Traditionally, this practice is done around midnight, but now everyone has different schedules, so adjust the practice to your life.

Take the same position as in the first practice, men on their right sides and women on their left. A particular form of breathing is to be done: inhale and hold the breath very gently. Lightly clench the perineum, the muscles of the floor of the pelvis, so that you have the sense of pulling the held breath upward. Try to experience the breath as being held just below the navel, compressed by the pressure from below. It is difficult to imagine this kind of breathing, and it may be necessary to experiment a bit until the sense of it is discovered. Better yet is to receive detailed instructions from a teacher.

After holding the breath for a few moments, gently exhale. During the exhalation, relax the muscles in the pelvis, the chest, and the whole body. Completely relax. Repeat this seven times.

The point of focus is the chakra centered slightly above and behind where the eyebrows would meet on the brow. Visualize a white, luminous ball of light (*tiglé**) in the chakra. It is a point of clarity. A tiglé, also known as *bindu*, can be many things, and is translated variously. In one context, it is an energetic quality that can be found in the body,

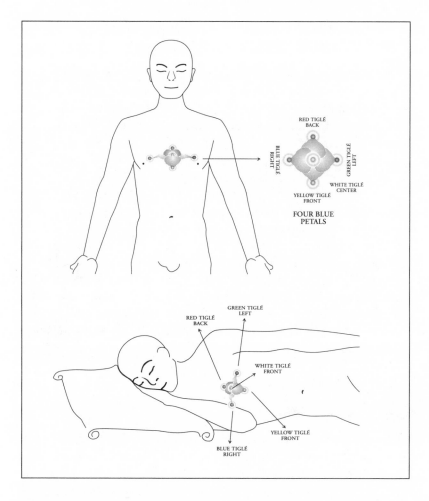

while in another context it can represent unbounded wholeness. As we use it in the practice, the tiglé is a small, insubstantial, luminous sphere of light. The different colored tiglés represent different qualities of consciousness and visualizing them is meant to act as a door into the experience of that quality.

The direction to "visualize" the tiglé does not mean you should picture a static image of a round white light; instead, imagine yourself merging with something really there. Try to feel the tiglé with your imaginal senses, and unify completely with it until only the clarity and luminosity exist. Some people will see the light clearly with their internal visual sense, while others will feel it more than see it. Feeling it is more important than seeing it. Most important is to merge with it entirely.

When connected with the luminous white tiglé in the brow chakra, the mind remains clear and present. As the experience of light increases, becoming more vivid and more inclusive, allow yourself to be absorbed in the light as the mind continues to increase in lucidity. If you sleep in this state, awareness becomes continuous. Developing clarity and continuity of presence is the purpose of this section of the practice. This is what is meant by "increasing the luminosity of dream." Try to connect with the sense behind the word "luminosity," to the actual experience. The metaphor only points to an experience that is deeper than language and visual representation.

Thus, "increasing" is what we call the quality of dreams manifested through this section of the practice. The sense here is of developing or growing toward completion, of generation, of bounty. The example given in the *Mother Tantra* is of a dream in which a dakini plays musical instruments, sings, and brings flowers, fruit, and clothing to the dreamer. Again, this does not mean that the dreams must include a dakini or any other specific image, but as the practitioner strengthens in this part of the practice, the dreams will be characterized by colorful enjoyment.

STRENTHENING PRESENCE

The third part of the practice is done roughly two hours after the second, about four hours into the sleep period. Traditionally, we think of this as two hours before dawn. For this part of the practice, a different

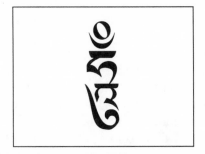

The Tibetan syllable HUNG

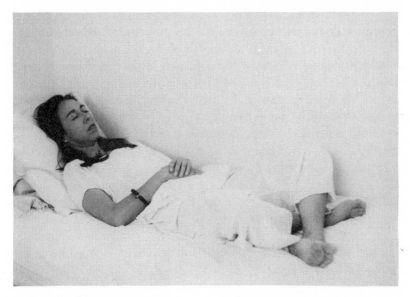

Reclining Meditation Posture

position is taken: Lay back on a high pillow. Cross the legs loosely, unlike in meditation posture; it does not matter whether the right or the left leg is on top. The position is somewhat similar to sleeping in a first class seat on an airplane: you recline but are not completely prone. Using a high pillow will help keep sleep light and generate more lucidity in dreams, but pay attention to the comfort of your neck. Do not remain in an uncomfortable position.

It is important to pay attention to the needs of the body. When I was a child I sat cross-legged in school for many hours each day, so this position is very easy for me. But it is different for most Westerners. The idea is not to endure pain all night, but to maintain continuity of awareness. Adjust the practice toward that goal.

For this part of the practice, take twenty-one deep, gentle breaths, maintaining full awareness of breathing.

The point of focus is the chakra of the heart, inside of which the black, luminous, syllable *HUNG* is visualized. It faces forward just as the body does. Merge with the syllable so that everything is the black *HUNG*. Become the black *HUNG*. Let the mind rest lightly in the black *HUNG*, and fall asleep.

The quality being developed here is power. You do not have to do anything; do not puff up to "try" to feel powerful. This is about finding the power you already have inside. The sense of power is also one of security; dreams generated in this part of the practice have to do with this sense of secure power. The examples in the *Mother Tantra* are dreams in which a powerful dakini directs the dreamer to sit on a throne, or the dreamer goes into a secure castle to receive teachings, or the dreamer is given approval by his or her father or mother. The quality is what is important, not the specific imagery. Instead of a dakini seating the dreamer on a throne, it may be the boss giving the dreamer a promotion, or the dreamer's mother organizing a party to celebrate the dreamer's accomplishments. Both dreams would be characteristic of this part of the practice. Rather than a castle, the dream may take place in a situation that makes the dreamer feel secure, and instead of a parent there may be another person in the dream who confers a sense of security, safety, and strength.

DEVELOPING FEARLESSNESS

The fourth part of the practice is the easiest because there is no need to wake again until morning. There is no particular position to take; just make yourself comfortable. There is no prescribed breathing; the breath is left in its natural rhythm. Traditionally this is two hours after the last waking, just before the light of dawn.

The "secret chakra" is the point of focus, the chakra behind the genitals. Inside the chakra is a sphere of black, luminous light: a black tiglé. This is the darker aspect of the imagination; the teaching says that dreams generated here are likely to contain wrathful dakinis, fire on the mountain and in the valleys, torrential rivers, or winds that destroy everything in their path. These are dreams in which the elements destroy the image of the self; the dreams can be terrifying. Discover if this is true for you. The quality of dreams in this section of the night should eventually become wrathful.

In this part of the practice, enter the black, luminous tiglé in the secret chakra and become it. Then let your mind relax and just lightly focus on the luminous black light that is everywhere, that pervades your senses and mind, and allow yourself to sleep.

The four qualities—peaceful, accomplishing, powerful, and wrathful—are very broad bands of associated images, feelings, emotions, and experiences. As stated above, it is not necessarily true that you will have the specific kinds of dreams presented as examples in the teachings. It is the quality that is the important point: the emotional timbre, the felt sense of the dream, the pervasive but possibly subtle currents in the experience of the dream. This is how to determine to which chakra the dream is connected, to which dimension of experience; it is not done by trying to decipher the dream contents. This also indicates where the prana and mind focus in the energetic system of the body to produce the specific dream. The dream may also be influenced by the events and experiences of the day that preceded it. By examining all that is connected to a dream, a great deal of information becomes available.

There is no further period of waking for practice, but of course you will wake again to start the day. When you do, try to wake in presence, in awareness of waking. The aim of the practice is to develop continuity of awareness through the night, across the periods of sleeping and waking, and during the whole day.

POSITION

Different body postures open or compress particular energetic channels and influence the flow of subtle energy. We use this understanding to aid specific processes in the practice. The Tibetan tradition considers the negative emotions to be more closely associated with the primary channel on the right side of the body in men and on the left in women. When a man sleeps on his right side, the channel that carries mostly negative prana is forced a little closed and the left channel opens. Also the lung, the physical organ, on that side is a bit compressed so the opposite lung is a little more responsible for the breath. You are probably already familiar with effects from lying on your side: when you lie on your right side you find it easier to breathe through your left nostril. For men, we consider this position beneficial to the movement of the positive wisdom prana through the left channel. Women benefit from the reverse, opening the wisdom channel that is on their right side by sleeping on their left. This affects dreams in a positive fashion and makes the dream practice easier. Opening the flow of the wisdom prana is a provisional expedient, as ultimately we want the balanced prana to move into the central channel.

Furthermore, by paying attention to posture, awareness is kept more stable during sleep. Where I come from, most people sleep on a three-foot by six-foot Tibetan carpet. If one moves too much, one falls out of bed. But that does not usually happen, because when one sleeps on something small, the position of the body is held in the sleeping mind throughout the night. For example, if one is sleeping on a narrow ledge, one maintains enough awareness to keep oneself from rolling off the edge. Here, in the big beds of the West, the sleeper can rotate like the hands of a clock and not fall, but holding the position anyway will help maintain awareness.

You can experiment with this when you find your concentration scattered. Change your position and calm and gentle the breath; you may find you can concentrate quite well. Breathing, the movement of prana, the position of the body, thoughts, and the quality of mind are all interrelated; unfolding this understanding allows the practitioner to consciously generate positive experiences.

FOCUSING THE MIND

Just as various body postures alter the flow of energy and affect the quality of experience, so do different visualizations focused in the body. Each of the four parts of the main practice involves focusing on a colored light and a tiglé or syllable in one of four chakras.

When we visualize a colored lotus, tiglé, or syllable at the site of a chakra, those things are not really there. The visualization is like a drawing or symbol representing the patterns and qualities of energy that move through that location. By using these images, the mind is better able to connect to the particular patterns of energy in their precise location in the body, and our consciousness is affected by that connection. Color also has an effect in consciousness, as we know from daily experience: if we enter a room painted all red our experience is quite different than if we enter a white room, a green room, or a black room. Color is used in visualization to help establish a particular quality in consciousness.

When we meditate, we tend to think of concentration and distraction as a switch that is either on or off, but this is not the case. Awareness can be focused in varying degrees of intensity. For example, when I came out of a long dark retreat, all visual phenomena were extremely intense. The houses and the trees, every color and every object, were vibrant. When I saw these same images every day they were unremarkable, but after fifty days of total darkness my focus on vision was so strong that everything was extraordinarily vivid. As the days went by, the visual phenomena seemed to dim, but of course the visual phenomena had not changed—it was my awareness of them that had diminished. Although the circumstances of my experience were unusual, they illustrate a general principle. All of our experiences will be more vivid if we have more intensity in the focus of our awareness.

In the practice, too, there are gradations in the level of focus. While just beginning the visualization at night there may be a very strong focus on the tiglé. As the body relaxes and sleep comes, the appearance of the visualization may weaken. The senses are fading and there is less hearing, smelling, touch, and so on. The fading of both the senses and the visualization is due to the focus of awareness diminishing in intensity and acuity. Next, there may be almost no feeling, another level of focus. Finally, there is no sensory experience at all and no image in the visualization.

It is difficult to notice these subtle distinctions, but they become apparent when more awareness is brought into the process of falling asleep. Even after the images and senses are completely dark, presence can be maintained. Eventually you will be able to go to sleep focusing on the *A* and then abide throughout the night in the pure presence the *A* represents. When you do, even the very first moments of waking in the morning will occur in pure presence.

You probably have already had experiences of maintaining a focus throughout the night. For example, when you need to wake for an early appointment, some awareness remains during sleep. Let's say you have to wake at five in the morning. You go to sleep but keep waking to check the clock. The awareness of the need to wake early remains although you are not strongly conceptualizing it, not thinking about it. The focus is very subtle. This is the kind of focus to bring to the practice, not strong concentration, but a light touch, gentle but consistent. If you are joyful before falling asleep because something wonderful has happened in your life, each time you wake, you wake to joy. It is continuous through sleep; you need not grimly hang on to it. Your awareness simply rests with it. This is the way to be with the tiglé: sleep with it as you sleep with joy.

There are two different relationships to phenomena relevant to focusing on the tiglé. In one, phenomena are grasped by the mind. In the other, phenomena appear to the mind. Grasping is a grosser form of dualistic interaction. The object is treated as an entity with inherent existence—as if it exists as a separate, distinct entity—and the mind holds onto it. When grasping ceases, it does not mean dualism is gone— phenomena still arise in experience and are conceptualized as separate entities—but the conceptualization is subtler. It might be said that the first is a more aggressive, active conceptualization, the second a more passive and weaker conceptualization. As it is weaker, it is also easier to dissolve in non-dual rigpa.

We begin the practice with the grosser form of dualism. Conceptualize the object and develop as strong an experience of it as possible using the imaginal senses: try to visualize it clearly and, even more importantly, feel it and let it affect the sensations in the body and energy, and the quality of the mind. After strongly establishing the object in awareness, loosen the focus. Let the object appear without effort, as if intention, lying below the surface of consciousness, binds the mind to the object, just as the mind stays connected to the need to wake for an early appointment or to a great joy. There is no need for exertion or concentration—the object just is and you are with it. You are no longer creating it, you are allowing it, observing it. It is similar to lying in the warm sun with closed eyes; without concentrating on the sun being "out there" you are warm, with the light, not separate from it. You do not have an experience of warmth and light—you need not try to keep your concentration on them—your experience *is* warmth and light, you are merged with it. This is how to be with the visualization during practice.

One common problem encountered in the beginning of practice is the disruption of sleep that occurs when the focus is held too tightly. The focus should be light: it is "being with" the tiglé rather than forcing the mind to be on it. The parallel to this in ordinary sleep is the difference between having images and thoughts drift through the mind as you fall asleep and being emotionally and intensely fixed on an object, which leads to insomnia. Let experience teach you; pay attention to what works and what does not, and adjust. If the practice keeps you awake, incrementally reduce the force of the focus until you can sleep.

Focusing on the tiglé or syllable, whether by grasping or by letting it appear, is only a first step. The real intent is to become unified with the object. Let us take, for example, the letter *A*. *A* is the symbol of the unborn, unchanging, natural state of mind; rather than focusing on it as an object, it is best to merge with the pervasive essence it represents. Actually this happens every night, because falling asleep is "falling" into pure rigpa, but when one is identified with the gross conceptual mind—which ceases functioning in deep sleep—the experience is of unconsciousness rather than rigpa. Rigpa can be discovered in sleep because it is already there.

Beyond letting the object appear to the mind, there is the non-dual state. The mind is still focused, but there is no identification with concepts, and thought is not used to visualize the tiglé or the *A*. The mind is simply present in awareness without division into subject and object. When there is focused awareness but no focuser and no object, you have the real sense of non-dual awareness. In the non-dual state, the *A* is not "there," and you are not "here." The image may or may not remain, but in either case, experience is not divided into subject and object. There is only the *A* and you are it. This is the significance of the clear *A* being tinged red by the light of the petals: you are to be the pure non-dual awareness symbolized by the *A* and, when experience arises, which is symbolized by the red of the petals, it colors the *A*, but the luminosity of non-dual presence is not lost.

Often practitioners say they have a hard time maintaining the visualization, or that the visualization interferes with sleep. Understanding this progression in the practice should clarify some of these issues. The progression is to see it, feel it, and then be it. When you fully merge with the object, the visualization may cease, and this is all right.

The teaching also prescribes this kind of focus at the time of death. When presence is maintained during death, the whole process is very different. Maintaining this presence is really the essence of the practice of the transference of consciousness at the time of death (*phowa*). In this practice, the intention is to move the mind directly into the pure space of awareness (*dharmakaya**). If successful, the practitioner does not experience the turbulence and distraction of the after-death experience but instead is liberated directly into the clear light.

Without the ability to remain in pure presence, we are distracted and wander off into dream, into fantasies, into samsara, into the next life, but if we maintain pure presence we find ourselves in the clear light during the night, we remain in the nature of mind during the day, and we are liberated in the bardo after death.

To experience how the visualizations affect consciousness try this: imagine being in total darkness, complete blackness. Not only is it dark around you, but it is dark in your vision, on your skin, above and below you, inside every cell of your body. It is almost as if you can feel, smell, and taste the darkness.

Now imagine the darkness suddenly giving way to clear, pervasive light all around you and in you, pervasive light that is you.

You should be able to feel the difference in these two visualizations through the subtle imaginal senses that illuminate your internal world, not just the visual aspect of the imagination. In the dark you have one experience, perhaps even a little fear or something wrathful, but in the light there is clarity.

Here is another experiment meant to give you some experience of the kind of focus the practice requires. Relax your body. Imagine a red, luminous *A* in your throat chakra. The red light is deep, rich, sensuous. Use your imagination to feel the light, let it calm you, relax you, quiet your mind and body, heal you. The light expands, filling your throat chakra and then your entire body. As it does, it relaxes every tension. Everything it touches dissolves into red light. Your entire body dissolves into red light. Let the light pervade your awareness so that all you see is luminous red light, all you feel is calm red light, any sound you hear is peaceful red light. Do not think this through—experience it. Let your mind be red light so that there is no you being aware of an object, only the red light being awareness itself. Allow whatever arises as subject or object to dissolve into red light. Everything—body and energy, world and mental events—dissolves until you are completely merged with red light. There is no "inside" or "outside," only red light. This is how to merge with the *A* and how to focus at night, unified with the object of the visualization.

THE SEQUENCE

The practices should always be done in order. The first part, focusing on the *A* in the throat, is done when first going to sleep. Ideally, the second part is done two hours later, the third two hours after that, and the fourth after two more hours. Waking throughout the night keeps the sleep lighter and makes it easier to accomplish dream yoga. It is not necessary to divide the night into exactly two-hour segments, although you can use an alarm clock if you wish; the point is simply to work with three periods of waking. We think in two-hour periods because people generally sleep for about eight hours. Although this schedule of waking will promote clarity, it is equally important to be rested, so do not worry if you miss one of the practice periods and just do three. Or even if you miss three and only do one. Do the best that you can, and anything that you cannot do, do not worry about. This is an important secret of practice! Worrying will not help your practice. But you also should not lose the force of your intention to do better. Just do the best you can.

So what do you do if after the first part you fall asleep and fail to wake again until dawn? Then practice the second part, not the third or fourth. Never skip one of the four primary practices. There is consistency in the results of the practice because all the elements are related: the different chakras, colors, meditations, times, elements, energies, and postures all work together to produce particular experiences and develop certain capacities in the practitioner. Each stage of the practice evokes a particular energetic quality of consciousness that is to be integrated with awareness, and each quality supports the development of the next. Because there is this kind of development, it is important that the four sessions be done in order.

The first part of the practice is imbued with the peaceful aspect of dreams. If you only do part of the practice, it is much easier to work with this peaceful aspect than, for example, the wrathful aspect. It is easier to stay present in a peaceful situation than a frightening one. It is a general principle of practice that we work more frequently with the situation that is easier to master and then practice with more difficult situations as we develop. In this case, we first develop stability in presence, and then work with more challenging aspects of experience: increasing clarity, developing power, and then the wrathful imagination.

The first part of the practice is not so much about trying to develop something as it is about rediscovering restful awareness. There is less trying to "do" and more allowing to "be." It is as if, after running around all day, you come home and relax into peaceful dreams. It takes a bit of time to rest up and be restored. The chakra used is the throat chakra, which is energetically connected to potentiality and expansion and contraction.

After two hours you wake. You should have gone deep enough into sleep to be rested and relaxed and this changes the attitude and quality of the mind. In the first session of practice, stability and focus are cultivated, which is like the base of the body. In the second session, you are to ornament the body, to develop clarity as an ornament of stabilized presence. Therefore, the focus is on the chakra in the brow, which is connected with opening and increasing clarity.

If stability is developed in the first session and clarity in the second, then power may be developed in the third. The focal point is the most central chakra in the body, the heart chakra, which is connected to the source of strength. This does not mean that just because you dream at this time you will have power in the dream. The power is developed as a result of the practice and the preceding two sessions. The power cultivated here is not a tough, aggressive power, but the power over thoughts and visions, the power to be free of habitual reactivity when encountering appearances. Like a king sitting on his throne—the seat of his power—you sit in the base of your power, in pure awareness.

In the fourth part of the night—based on stability, clarity, and power—fearlessness is developed. We have in us the causes for frightening dreams and, after some accomplishment in the first three stages of the practice, we call them out by focusing on the black tiglé in the secret chakra, the chakra most connected to wrathful karmic traces. The generation of frightening dreams is, here, a result of practice and the practitioner is encouraged to continue dreams of this kind, to use the practice to transform even frightening karmic traces into the path. We test our development in the practice in this way and further strengthen the stability, clarity, and power we have cultivated. Terrifying images no longer produce fearful emotions but are welcomed as opportunities for developing the practice.

There is one alternative: you may, if you wish, focus on only one point of the practice until the appropriate results are attained. The practices must still be done in order, but in this case you work with just the first section of the practice every time you wake, repeating it many times over many days, until you have experience in generating peaceful dreams and stability of awareness. After there is some accomplishment in the first part, you may work only with the second, increasing clarity, for as many nights as it takes to generate dreams that are of the quality of this section of the practice and until there is some increase in clarity during the night. Then practice the third until the results manifest, and finally practice the fourth. But do not do the second part if you have not done the first, or the fourth if you have not done the third. To reiterate: the sequence is important.

Some people will feel overwhelmed by the seeming complexity of the practice, but it only appears this way in the beginning. As dream yoga is mastered, the practice becomes simpler and simpler. When awareness is stable, one need not do any of the particular forms of the practice. It is enough just to abide in presence and dreams will naturally be lucid. The practice only appears to be complex because a number of different elements are working in harmony to best support the practitioner, and it is particularly in the beginning of the practice that we need the most support. Take the time to fully understand each element in the preparations and the practices and use them together. Once you are consistently lucid in dream, you can experiment with simplifying the practice.

6 Lucidity

If someone tells us they spent many years in retreat we are impressed, and rightly so; this kind of effort is needed to attain enlightenment. But in our busy lives such a thing may seem to be impossible. We may wish to do a traditional three-year retreat but feel that our circumstances will never allow it. But actually, we all have the possibility of doing this much practice. During the next ten years of life we will spend over three years in sleep. In ordinary dreams we may have lovely experiences, but we may also practice anger or jealousy or fear. Perhaps these are emotional experiences we need to have, but we do not need to continue in such a way that we increase the habitual inclination to be attached to and overwhelmed by emotions and fantasies. Why not practice the path instead? Those three years of sleep can be spent doing the practices. Once lucidity is stabilized, any practice can be done in dream, some more effectively and with more consequence than when they are done during the day.

Dream yoga develops the capacity that we all have for lucid dreaming. A lucid dream, in this context, is one in which the dreamer is aware during the dream that he or she is dreaming. Many people, perhaps most people, have had at least one experience of lucid dreaming. It may have been in a nightmare in which one realized that one was in a dream and woke to escape. Or it may just have been an unusual experience. Some people regularly have lucid dreams without any conscious intention to do so. As the preliminary and main practices are integrated into the life of the practitioner, lucid dreams will begin to occur with increasing frequency. Lucid dreaming is not in itself the goal of practice, but it is an important development along the path of this yoga.

There are many different levels of lucid dreaming. At the superficial level, one may realize that one is in a dream but have little clarity and no power to affect the dream. Lucidity is found and then lost, and the logic of the dream prevails over the conscious intent of the dreamer. At the other end of the continuum, lucid dreams can be extraordinarily vivid, seemingly "realer" than ordinary waking experience. With experience, greater freedom is developed in the dream and the boundaries of the mind are overcome, until one can do literally anything that one can think of to do.

Obviously, dreams do not occur in the same dimension of reality as waking life. Getting a new car in dream does not mean that you will not have to take the bus to work in the morning. In this sense, we may find dreams unsatisfactory: we feel they are not "real." However, in accomplishing psychological tasks that are incomplete, or overcoming energetic difficulties, the effects of the dream can extend into waking life. Most importantly, in dream the mind's limitations can be challenged and overcome. As they are, we develop flexibility of mind, and this is most important.

Why is flexibility of mind so important? Because the rigidities of mind, the limitations of wrong views that obscure wisdom and constrict experience, keep us ensnared in illusory identities and prevent us from finding freedom. Throughout this book I emphasize how ignorance, grasping, and aversion condition us and keep us trapped in negative karmic tendencies. To progress on the spiritual path we must lessen grasping and aversion until we can penetrate the ignorance at their base and discover the wisdom behind it. Flexibility of the mind is the capacity that, when it is developed, allows us to overcome grasping and aversion. It allows us to see things in a new way and respond positively rather than being driven blindly by habitual reactions.

Different people sharing the same situation react differently. Some grasp more and some less. The more grasping there is—the more reacting from karmic conditioning—the more we are controlled by experiences we encounter. With enough flexibility, we are not driven by karma. A mirror does not choose what to reflect; everything is welcome to come and go in its pure nature. The mirror, in this sense, is flexible, and it is so because it neither grasps nor pushes away. It does not try to hold on to one reflection and refuse to allow another. We lack this flexibility because we do not understand that whatever appears in awareness is only the reflection of our own mind.

In lucid dreams, we practice transforming whatever is encountered. There is no boundary to experience that cannot be broken in dream; we can do whatever occurs to us to do. As we break habitual limitations of experience, the mind becomes increasingly supple and flexible. First we develop lucidity and then flexibility, and then we apply this flexibility of mind to all of our life. We are less inhibited by our habitual identities when we have the experience of transforming them and letting them go. We are less constricted by our habitual perceptions when we have experience of their relativity and malleability.

Just as dream images can be transformed in dream, so emotional states and conceptual limitations can be transformed in waking life. With experience of the dreamy and malleable nature of experience, we can transform depression into happiness, fear into courage, anger into love, hopelessness into faith, distraction into presence. What is unwholesome we can change to wholesome. What is dark we can change to light. What is restricted and solid we can change into the open and spacious. Challenge the boundaries that constrict you. The purpose of these practices is to integrate lucidity and flexibility with every moment of life, and to let go of the heavily conditioned way we have of ordering reality, of making meaning, and of being trapped in delusion.

DEVELOPING FLEXIBILITY

The teachings suggest many things to do in dreams after lucidity has been developed. The first step in developing flexibility in dream, as in waking, is to recognize the potential for doing so. As we think about the possibilities the teachings suggest, the mind incorporates them into its potential. We become capable of experiences we could not even conceptualize before.

I have a laptop computer that is a lot of fun to explore. If I click on one of the icons on the screen, a file opens. Click on another, and something else appears on the screen. The mind is like that. The attention goes to something and it is like clicking on an icon; suddenly a train of thought and images appear. The mind keeps clicking, moving from one thing to another. Sometimes we have two windows open, as when we are talking to someone and also thinking about something else.

While ordinarily we do not think of this as having multiple selves or multiple identities, we can manifest those multiple selves in a dream. Rather than simply having our attention divided, in dream we can divide into different, simultaneously existing dream bodies.

After playing with my computer one day, I dreamt I was looking at a screen upon which icons would appear that I could click on with my mind, changing the whole environment. An icon for forest appeared and when I clicked on it I was in a forest. Then an icon for ocean, and after clicking on it, I was suddenly in an ocean setting. The capacity to do this was already in my mind, but the way that it arose as a possibility for experience came from interacting with my computer. Our thoughts and experiences influence further thoughts and experiences. Dream practice works with this fact. The teachings present us with new ideas, new possibilities, and the tools to realize those possibilities, and then it is up to us to manifest them in dreams and waking life.

For instance, the teachings talk about multiplying things in dream. Perhaps we dream of three flowers. Because we are aware of being in a dream and the flexibility of dream, if we wish we can make a hundred flowers, a thousand flowers, a rain of flowers. But first we need to recognize the possibility. If we do not know this kind of multiplication of objects is an option, then, for us, the option does not exist.

Research with dreams in the West has found that people can improve skills by practicing them in dreams and daydreams. Centuries ago, this understanding was incorporated in the teachings. Using dreams, we can decrease the negative and increase the positive, changing our habitual ways of being in the world. And this need not be directed only to skills that will aid us in daily life, but can also be applied at the most profound levels of the spiritual life. Always aim for the highest, most inclusive goal, as this will automatically take care of the lesser. While it is good to work on relative issues, after enlightenment there are no problems at all.

The *Mother Tantra* lists eleven categories of experience in which the mind is usually bound by appearance. All of these are to be recognized, challenged, and transformed. The principle is the same in all, but it is helpful to spend time thinking about each to introduce the possibilities of transformation to your own mind. The categories are: size; quantity; quality; speed; accomplishment; transformation; emanation; journey; seeing; encounter; and experiences.

Size. We seldom think much about size in our dreams, but we do in our waking life. There are two aspects of size, smaller and larger. Change your size in the dream, become as small as an insect and then as large as a mountain. Take a big problem and make it small. Take a small, beautiful flower and make it as large as the sun.

Quantity. If there is one buddha in your dream, increase the number to one hundred or one thousand. And if there are one thousand problems, make them one. In dream practice, you can burn the seeds of incipient karma. Using awareness, drive the dream rather than be driven; dream rather than let yourself be dreamt.

Quality. When people get stuck in an unwholesome experience, it is often because they do not know that it can be changed. You must think about the possibility of change, and then practice it in the dream. When you are angry in a dream, change that emotion to love. You can change the qualities of fear, jealousy, anger, greed, incessant hopefulness, and dullness. None of these is helpful. Tell yourself that they can be overcome by transforming them. You can even say this out loud in order to strengthen your knowing. Once you have the experience of changing emotion in dream, you can have it in waking life, too. This is developing freedom and flexibility; you do not have to be trapped by prior conditioning.

Speed. In just a few seconds of dream, many things can be accomplished, because you are entirely in the mind. Slow down an experience until each moment is a whole world. Visit a hundred places in a minute. The only boundaries in a dream are the boundaries in your imagination.

Accomplishment. Whatever you have been unable to accomplish in life, you can accomplish in dream. Do practices, write a book, swim across an ocean, finish what needs finishing.

A year after my mother passed away, she appeared in my dream and asked for help. I asked her what I could do. She gave me a drawing of a stupa and asked that I build it for her. I knew I was dreaming, but I accepted the task as if it were real. I was in Italy at the time, where there are many building restrictions and zoning laws. I did not know how to get the permits, the money, and the land that I needed. So I thought to ask my guardians. This is what the *Mother Tantra* recommends: ask the dream guardians for help when confronted with a task that it seems you cannot accomplish.

In response to my request for help, the guardians appeared. A giant bodhi tree stood in the dream and suddenly the guardians turned it into the stupa. In our culture, we believe that building a stupa for someone who has died helps that person to go on to their next birth. My mother was happy and satisfied in the dream, and so was I. I felt that I had given something important to her, something that perhaps had not happened at home in India when she died. Now it was accomplished and my mother and I were both happy. The feeling carried over into my waking life.

The accomplishments in dream influence waking life. By working with experience, you work with the karmic traces. Use the dream to accomplish what is important to you.

Transformation. Transformation is very important for practitioners of tantra, as it is the principle underlying tantric practice, but it is also important for all of us. Learn to transform yourself. Try everything. Transform yourself into a bird, a dog, a garuda, a lion, a dragon. Transform yourself from an angry person into a compassionate person, from a grasping, jealous human into an open, clear buddha. Transform yourself into the yidam and into the dakini. This is very powerful for developing flexibility and overcoming the limitations of your habitual identities.

Emanation. This is similar to transformation. After transforming yourself into a yidam or a buddha, emanate many more bodies that can be of benefit to other beings. Be in two bodies, then three, four, as many as you can, and then more. Break through the limitation of experiencing yourself as a single, separate ego.

Journey. Start with places that you wish to go. You want to go to Tibet? Take a trip there. To Paris? Go. Where have you always wanted to go?

This is not the same as simply arriving somewhere, this is about the journey. Guide yourself there consciously. You can travel to another country or to a pure land where there is no defilement. Or travel to another planet, or a place you have not seen in many years, or to the bottom of the ocean.

Seeing. Try to see what you have not seen before. Have you ever seen Guru Rinpoche? Tapihritsa? Christ? Now you can. Have you seen Shambhala or the center of the sun? Have you seen cells dividing or your heart pumping or the top of Mt. Everest or the view from a bee's eye? Generate ideas for yourself and then make them real in dream.

Encounter. In the Tibetan tradition, there are many stories of people meeting teachers and guardians and dakinis and so on in their dreams. Maybe you feel a connection to teachers of the past; now meet them. When you do, right away ask if you can meet a second time. That creates more of an opportunity to meet them again. Then ask for teachings.

Experience. Use the dream to experience something you have not done yet. If you are uncertain about your experience of rigpa, then have it in the dream. You can experience any mystic state or experience of the path, however elaborate or simple. You can breathe water like a fish, or walk through walls, or become a cloud. You can travel the universe as a beam of light or fall as rain from the sky. Whatever you can think of, you can do.

Go beyond the limits of the above categories; they are only suggestions. We work with patterns in our experience—like speed, size, emanation, and so on—because we get stuck believing in the reality of these relative concepts. Dissolving boundaries in the mind leads us toward the freedom that is the base of the mind. If you dream of a threatening fire, transform yourself into flame; of a flood, transform yourself into water. If a demon chases you, transform into a bigger demon. Become a mountain, a leopard, a redwood tree. Become a star or an entire forest. Transform yourself from a man into a woman, and then into a hundred women. Or transform yourself from a woman into a goddess. Transform into animals, a hawk flying far above the ground, or a spider weaving a web. Transform into a bodhisattva and manifest yourself in a hundred places at the same time, or in all thirty-three hells, to benefit the beings there. Transform into Siamuhka, into Padmasambhava, or any other deity, yidam, or dakini. This practice is the same as those tantric practices in which you transform yourself. It has the same goals and reasons, but it is much easier to accomplish in a dream; you actually transform. Infinite experiences of transformation are available in dream.

Travel anywhere you have ever wanted to go: to Mount Meru, the center of the earth, other planets, other realms. Almost every night I go back to India—a very cheap way to travel. Go to the realms of the gods. Travel in hell, in the devil realm. It is just an idea, you will not actually be participating there. But you will be loosening the constrictions that bind your mind.

Participate in the practices and pujas of the gods and goddesses. Participate with the five buddha families. Fly through the ground. Travel through the inside of your own body. Make yourself as big as the earth, then bigger. Or as small as an atom, as thin as a bamboo, as light as floating pollen.

The principle of developing flexibility is more important than the particulars of the dream, just as the luminous quality of the crystal is more important than the color of light it happens to be reflecting. The suggestions from the teachings should not become more limits. Think up new possibilities and manifest them, until whatever seems to limit your experience is immediately seen to be fragile and non-binding. Lucidity brings more light to the conceptual mind, and exercising flexibility loosens the knots of conditioning that constrict it. As we are conditioned by the apparently solid entities we encounter, they should be transformed in our experience, made luminous and transparent. As we are conditioned by the apparent solidity of thoughts, they should be dissolved in the limitless freedom of the mind.

There is a basic principle for the spiritual journey that we should continue to exercise even in the freedom of the dream. The possibilities in dream are unlimited, we can make whatever changes to the dream that we wish, but it is still important that we change toward the positive. That is the direction that will best serve our spiritual path. Actions taken in dream have an effect in us internally just as actions taken in waking life. There is tremendous freedom in dream but there is no freedom from karmic cause and effect until we are free of dualism. We need patience and strong intention to develop the flexibility necessary to overthrow the dictates of negative karma.

Work at the boundaries of experience, the constrictions of conditioning and limiting beliefs. The mind is amazing: it can do this. Your identity is more flexible than you can imagine. You simply need to be aware of the possibility of changing experience and identity and then it is a real possibility. If you believe that you cannot do something, then usually you cannot. It is a very simple point and one that is very important. The moment you say you can do something you have already begun.

Treat your dreams with respect and incorporate all of the experiences of the dream, like your waking life, into the path. Using the dream to develop freedom from limitations, to overcome obstacles in your path, and finally to recognize your true nature and the true nature of all phenomena, is to use the dream wisely.

7 The Obstacles

The *Mother Tantra* describes four obstacles that may be encountered in dream yoga: distraction in delusive fantasy, laxity, restlessness that results in waking, and forgetting. It prescribes both internal and external remedies.

DELUSION

Distraction by delusion occurs when an external or internal sound or image carries the attention away. Perhaps there is a sound from outside as the practitioner is falling asleep. The mind moves toward it and then, through association, a memory or fantasy may arise and the practitioner becomes entangled in it with a corresponding emotional reaction. Or the sound may generate curiosity and the practitioner becomes lost in speculation. This is delusion, because we are caught up in chasing after things that do not actually exist in the way we think of them.

The internal antidote is to focus on the central channel. What does this feel like? Try it—you will find that you feel centered and present, you come out of fantasy and back to yourself. It is helpful to fall asleep with awareness of the central channel. Be simple in this. We sometimes get so intense about practices that we make them needlessly complex. Just feel the central channel; this will prevent the mind from running away. It is also helpful to meditate on impermanence and the illusory nature of our dualistic experience, as these contemplations will strengthen the intention to remain focused and avoid becoming lost in fantasy. The external antidote is to make an offering or do devotional practices like guru yoga.

LAXITY

The second obstacle is laxity. It manifests as an internal laziness, a lack of internal strength and clarity. When you are lax in practice, you drift around, clouded and perhaps comfortable, even while attending to the object of attention. This is different than the first obstacle, in which your attention chases a distraction. In this case there is a lack of internal sharpness.

The antidote is to visualize blue smoke slowly drifting up the central channel from the junction of the three channels (a few inches below the navel and in the center of the body) to the throat. Do not get hung up thinking of physics—where the smoke goes and if it collects and that kind of thing. Just visualize the smoke slowly moving up the central channel, as if it were already a dream. Besides doing this, you may visit your teacher or a healer and ask for something like an exorcism. The *Mother Tantra* suggests that when laxity occurs you may be encountering a problem with a spirit or with a force in your environment, although this is certainly not the only way to understand the difficulty.

SELF-DISTRACTION

The third obstacle is self-distraction. You wake again and again and are restless in sleep. The cause may be a problem with the prana, or you may be excited or agitated. The antidote is to focus on four dakinis in the form of four syllables which rest on the four petals of a lotus in the throat chakra. The syllables are *RA*, which is yellow and is toward the front of your body. *LA*, which is green, is to your left. *SHA*, to the back, is red. And *SA* is to the right and is blue. If there is a problem with restless self-distraction, focus on the syllables one after the other as you fall asleep. Try to feel protector dakinis in all directions. Externally, doing the chöd practice, a ritual that involves making offerings to spirits, can be of benefit. Also, determine if you have broken commitments (*samaya**) that you may have made involving the teaching or your teacher. Relationships with friends or acquaintances that are disturbed can also cause this restlessness. Self-confession can be useful.

To do this, visualize your teacher as in guru yoga, and confess what is wrong. Examine it, not with guilt or shame or any other bad feeling, but with awareness. If you did something that was not right, decide not to do it again. Perhaps there is also some action that should be taken, such as talking with the friend with whom you are disturbed; you can decide to take such an action.

FORGETTING

The fourth obstacle is forgetting—forgetting your dreams and to do the practice. Even if you have helpful experiences they may be forgotten. Doing a personal retreat can help by bringing more clarity to the mind. Balancing the prana using the breath can settle and steady the awareness. The *Mother Tantra* prescribes the practice of the first watch of the night as an antidote; this is the first primary practice, described earlier, focusing on the red *A* at the throat. Keep awareness on the *A* while falling asleep and this will help you remember.

FOUR OBSTACLES ACCORDING TO SHARDZA RINPOCHE

Shardza Rinpoche also writes of four possible obstacles, but categorizes them differently: problems with prana, mind, local spirits, and illness. These obstacles can prevent you from having or remembering dreams as well as create problems in the dream itself.

If you suffer from a problem of prana, the energy in the body is blocked or is in some way prevented from circulating smoothly. The mind and the prana are connected; if the prana is disturbed the mind will be also. In this case, anything that will help you relax before bed, like a massage or hot bath, is an aid. Also, try to remain as calm and relaxed as possible during the day.

The mind can be too busy to allow sleep. For example, after a very hectic day it is sometimes hard to stop thinking about it—your mind is spread out over problems or excitements and is tight with intensity or anxiety. If you find it difficult to calm the mind, it is sometimes helpful to do hard physical work, to tire the body or even exhaust it. Meditating on emptiness can also clear the mind. And, as above, taking whatever steps you can to relax before sleep is helpful.

A disturbance with the local spirits can result in broken and unrestful sleep. I know that many Westerners do not believe in such things—that the local spirits are actually the energy of the place or the feel of the environment—and in a way they are right. But Tibetans believe that there really are spirits, beings living in a locale, and if one does something that energetically interferes with those beings, one can be affected by them in return. The provocation of local spirits may result in terrible dreams, or the inability to remember dreams, or in restlessness that prevents sleep.

In this situation we first need to become aware of the nature of the problem. For Tibetans there are several remedies for this kind of disturbance. They often go to a shaman and ask for divination in order to discover the source of the problem and an appropriate action to take. Or they may do chöd practice, making offerings to the spirits. Or they will go to the master and ask for help that is usually given in the form of something like an exorcism, a ritual that severs the spirit's connection to them. If the master does this, he will usually ask for something belonging to the petitioner, a few hairs or an article of clothing, and burn it in the ritual fire. Tibetans have many remedies like this, but they are only of benefit if you understand the problem and believe that the spirits are provoking you so that you take the steps necessary to repair the situation. If you do have experience of spirits in this fashion, offer them compassion. If you do not believe in such things but are sensitive to the energy of the place, correct it by burning incense and generating compassion. And if you do not believe in this either, generate compassion to change the internal environment of your mind and emotions.

The fourth obstacle is illness and the teaching recommends, of course, that you go to a doctor.

There is no obstacle you will encounter that has not been encountered and overcome by others before you, so you need not become discouraged. Rely on the teachings and your teacher to discover the remedies, which exist in the teachings and only need to learned and applied.

8 Controlling and Respecting Dreams

Some schools of Western psychology believe it is harmful to control dreams, that dreams are a regulatory function of the unconscious or a form of communication between parts of ourselves that should not be disturbed. This view suggests that the unconscious exists and that it is a repository of experience and meaning. The unconscious is thought to form the dream and embed in it meaning that will either be explicit and obvious or latent and in need of interpretation. In this context, the self is often thought to be composed of the unconscious and conscious aspects of the individual, and the dream is thought to be a necessary medium of communication between the two. The conscious self can then benefit by working with the dream, mining it for the meaning and insight that the unconscious has placed in it. Or it may benefit from the catharsis of the dream or from the balancing of physiological processes through the dream-making activity.

Understanding emptiness radically changes our understanding of the dreaming process. These three entities—the unconscious, the meaning, and the conscious self—are all entities that exist only through imputing reality to that which by itself has none. It is important to understand what is being said here. The concern that the encroachment of the conscious mind upon the unconscious is damaging to natural processes makes sense if you posit the elements of the situation as discrete elements of the individual, working in cooperation with one another. But this view understands only one dimension of the individual's internal dynamics, often to the detriment of a more expansive identity.

As mentioned earlier, there are two levels of working with dreams. One involves finding meaning in the dream. This is good, and it is the level of most of the Western psychologies that accord value to dreams. In both the East and the West, it is understood that dreams can be a source of creativity, solutions to problems, diagnosis of ills, and so on. But the meaning in dreams is not inherent to the dream; it is being projected onto the dream by the individual examining the dream and then is "read" from the dream. The process is much like describing the images that seem to appear in the ink-spot tests used by some psychologists. The meaning does not exist independently. Meaning does not exist until someone starts to look for it. Our mistake is that rather than seeing the truth of the situation, we begin to think that there really is an unconscious, a thing, and that the dream is real, like a scroll with a secret message written on it in code that, if cracked, anyone could read.

We need a deeper understanding of what the dream is, of what experience is, to truly utilize dreaming as an approach to enlightenment. When we practice deeply, many wonderful dreams will arise, rich with signs of progress. But ultimately the meaning in the dream is not important. It is best not to regard the dream as correspondence from another entity to you, not even from another part of you that you do not know. There is no conventional meaning outside of the dualism of samsara. This view is not a giving in to chaos: there is no chaos or meaninglessness either, these are more concepts. It may sound strange, but this idea of meaning must be abandoned before the mind can find complete liberation. And doing this is the essential purpose of dream practice.

We do not ignore the use of the meaning in dreaming. But it is good to recognize that there is also dreaming in meaning. Why expect great messages from a dream? Instead penetrate to what is below meaning, the pure base of experience. This is the higher dream practice—not psychological, but more spiritual—concerned with recognizing and realizing the fundament of experience, the unconditioned. When you progress to this point, you are unaffected by whether there is a message in the dream or not. Then you are complete, your experience is complete, you are free from the conditioning that arises from dualistic interactions with the projections of your own mind.

Most of dream practice is done while the practitioner is awake in order to influence the dream. It is not about directly controlling the dream. The aspect of directly controlling the dream, and the one that more people may be concerned about, occurs during lucid dream. Multiplying yourself in a dream is an example, as is transforming or creating dream entities. The teaching says that doing this is a very good thing, as the capacity to do these things means that flexibility of the mind is being developed. Furthermore, the same kind of flexibility and control is to be brought into waking life; not in order to fly, but to understand the constructed nature of experience and the freedom inherent in that understanding. Rather than being controlled by feelings, you can change yourself and the story that you tell about yourself, and do what is truly important rather than remaining stuck in a nightmare or an endlessly shifting dream or even a pleasant fantasy.

It is not different than waking life. Karmic traces cause dreams, and our reactions to experience create further karmic traces. During a dream these dynamics are still in effect. We do want to control our dreams rather than being controlled by them, just as during the day it is better not to be controlled by thoughts or emotions but to respond to situations fully from our awareness.

We want to influence our dreams. We want them to be clearer and more integrated with our practice, just as we should want these qualities for every moment of our life. There is no danger in this of disrupting something important. All we disrupt is our ignorance.

9 Simple Practices

Accomplishment of dream and sleep yogas depends on the individual's faith, intention, commitment, and patience. There is no single practice that will accomplish realization in one night's efforts. Spiritual maturation takes time, and it is in time that we live out our ordinary lives. When we fight time, we lose. But when we know how to be in time, the practice spontaneously unfolds by itself.

The entirety of dream yoga may seem too complex and require too much to become a reality in our life. But there is much we can do, adding a little here and there, integrating it into our life, until gradually we make our entire life into practice. Here are things that anyone can do that will lead to success in dream yoga.

THE WAKING MIND

The waking part of the day is around sixteen hours, and the mind is busy the whole time. Often, it seems there is not enough time, and so much of what time there is, is spent in distraction and unpleasant experience. The modern world seems constantly to be making demands—to take care of job and family, to watch movies, to look in store windows, to wait in traffic, to talk to friends—a thousand things to grab attention and carry it off, until the day is a blur leading to exhaustion and the hunger for even greater distraction that offers escape. Moment by moment we are driven away from ourselves. Living this way is not helpful for any practice, including dream yoga. Therefore, simple and regular habits of reconnecting to ourselves, of becoming more present, must be cultivated.

Every breath can be a practice. With the inhalation, imagine drawing in pure, cleansing, relaxing energies. And with each exhalation, imagine expelling all obstacles, stress, and negative emotions. This is not something that requires a particular place in which to sit. It can be done when in the car on the way to work, waiting for a stop light, sitting in front of the computer, preparing a meal, cleaning the house, or walking.

A powerful but simple practice is to try to maintain presence in the body continuously throughout the day. Feel the body as a whole. The mind is worse than a crazed monkey, jumping from one thing to the next; it has a hard time focusing on one thing. But the body is a source of experience more stable and constant, and using it as an anchor for awareness will help the mind to grow calmer and more focused. Just as the participation of the mind is essential in organizing and nourishing the physical aspects of life, the mind needs the body in order to stabilize in calm presence, which is fundamentally important to all practices.

For example, while walking in a park the body may be in the park while the mind is off working in the office, or at home, or talking to a distant friend, or making a list of groceries. That means the mind has disconnected from the body. Instead, when looking at a flower, really look at it. Be fully present. With the help of the flower, bring the mind back to the park. Appreciation for sensory experience reconnects mind and body. When the experience of the flower is felt throughout the body, a healing occurs; this can be the same when seeing a tree, smelling smoke, feeling the cloth of your shirt, hearing a bird call, or tasting an apple. Train yourself to vividly experience sensory objects without judgement. Try completely to be the eye with form, the nose with smell, the ear with sound, and so on. Try to be complete in experience while remaining in just the bare awareness of the sensory object.

When this ability is developed, reactions will still occur. Upon seeing the flower, judgements about its beauty will arise, or a smell may be judged to be foul. Even so, with practice the connection to the pure sensory experience can be maintained rather than continuing to become lost in the mind's distraction. Being distracted by a cloud of concepts is a habit and it can be replaced with a new habit: using bodily sensual experience to bring us to presence, to connect us to the beauty of the world, to the vivid and nourishing experience of life that lies under our distractions. This is the underpinning of successful dream yoga.

The first moment of perception is always clear and bright. It is only the distraction of the mind that prevents us from recognizing this and experiencing each moment of life with appreciation. Relying on this practice uses the steadiness of form and the vivid sensual experience of the sensory world to support those qualities of the mind most conducive to successful dream practice.

PREPARING FOR NIGHT

Often we feel half-dead after a stressful day. Then we fall into bed and become almost completely dead. We do not even spend a few minutes to connect body and mind in presence, but spend the evening in distraction and remain in distraction as we prepare for bed and as we drift away in sleep. Connecting mind, body, and feeling is one of the most important things that we can do to insure our progression on the spiritual path. We should take a little time to do that each night before sleep.

When we fall asleep with mind and body disconnected, they each go their own way. The body holds on to stress and tensions accumulated during the day, and the mind, too, continues as it was during the day, running from one place to another, one time to another, ungrounded and lacking any steadiness and calm. It exists in an anxious or drowsy state, with little presence. In this situation, we lack power and awareness, and dream yoga becomes very difficult.

To change this situation, to have healthier sleep and stronger results in dream practice, spend a few minutes before sleep reconnecting to presence and calm. Simple things are effective: take a bath, burn a candle and incense, sit in front of a shrine or even in your bed and connect with enlightened beings or your master. You can generate feelings of compassion, pay attention to the feeling of your body, and cultivate the experiences of joy, happiness, and gratitude. Generating positive thoughts and feelings, fall asleep. The prayers and the love will relax the body and gentle the mind, and bring joy and peace to both. As suggested earlier, imagine being surrounded by enlightened protective beings, particularly by dakinis. Imagine them protecting you as a mother does her child, radiating love and compassion toward you. Then, feeling secure and at peace, pray, "May I have a clear dream. May I have a lucid dream. May I understand myself through dream." Repeat these lines again and again, out loud or internally. This is so simple to do, but it will change the quality of sleep and dreams and you will be more rested and grounded in the morning.

If you feel that the four stages of practice are too complicated—the focus on the throat, brow, heart, and secret chakra—just focus on the throat chakra. Imagine a red, luminous *A* there, after you have prayed. Focus on it, feel it, and fall asleep. It is important to have calmed yourself beforehand, to feel connected to the body. If even the concentration on the *A* seems too difficult or complex, then just feel your entire body, and connect to presence and to compassion. This is the way to clean the mind and the body, which have become stressed and foggy during the day. Every night we brush our teeth and wash, and we feel better and sleep better. If instead we go to sleep feeling dirty and unclean, our sleep and dreams are affected. We all know this about the physical level of our existence, but we often forget how important it is to feel that freshness and connectedness in our mind, too. Maybe we should write a sentence on our toothbrushes, "After this, wash your mind."

You can also work with breathing as you go to sleep. Try to breathe equally in both nostrils. If the right is blocked, sleep on your left side and vice versa. Gentle the breath and allow it to be smooth and quiet. As suggested earlier, exhale stress and negative emotion, inhale pure healing energy. Do this breath nine times, in meditation posture or while lying down, then focus on the red *A* in the throat. Feel the *A* rather than focus on it, merge with it rather than remain separate from it. Upon waking, if you find you feel better and more rested, feel good about your success. Feel the blessings of the masters and the enlightened beings, the pleasure of your own joyful efforts, and the happiness of following the spiritual path. That happiness will encourage the next night's practice and aid in sustaining and developing the practice continuously.

It is not unusual to find it difficult to relax or to feel compassion or love when going to sleep. If you are in this situation, use your creative imagination. Imagine lying on a beautiful, warm beach or walking in clean, fresh mountain air. Imagine those things that make you feel relaxed, rather than simply falling down into sleep, driven out of presence by the emotions and stresses of the day. Even these simple practices will be of great help.

10 Integration

Dream practice is not just for personal growth or to generate interesting experiences. It is part of the spiritual path and its results should affect all aspects of life by changing the practitioner's identity and the relationship between the practitioner and the world. Most of what is included in this section on integrating the dream practice with the life of the practitioner has already been mentioned, but here it is summarized.

There are two general stages of dream practice: the conventional and the non-conventional, or the dualistic and non-dual. We have primarily focused on the first, which is connected with working with dream images and stories, with our responses to experience and our emotions, with dream's effects in us and the effects of our practice in dream, and with developing greater awareness and control.

The non-conventional level of practice involves neither the content of dreams nor our experiences of them, but rather the non-dual clear light. This is the final goal of dream practice and of sleep practice.

We should never disparage the dualistic use of dream yoga. After all, for most of us, and most of the time, we live in the world of duality and it is in our ordinary life that we must travel our spiritual path. Working with dream practices, we transform anger to love, hopelessness to hopefulness, what is wounded in us to what is healed and strong. We develop the ability to work skillfully with the situations in life and to be of aid to others. We gain these skills when we begin to truly understand that life is dreamlike and flexible. Then we can change ordinary life into experiences of great beauty and meaningfulness, incorporating everything into the path.

It is only when our conventional selves dissolve into rigpa that we truly move beyond the need for hope and meaning, beyond the discriminations of positive and negative. The non-conventional truth is beyond healing and the need for healing. To assume this perspective while we are not actually living in the non-dual view leads to a kind of muddled spirituality in which we exercise our negative conditioning and think that we are exercising freedom. When we abide fully in the clear light, negativities no longer rule us, so it is easy to test ourselves and see if we are there or not.

There are four successive domains of integration related to dream practice: vision, dream, bardo, and clear light. Vision here means all experiences of waking life, including all that is encountered with the senses and all internal events. Vision is integrated into dream when all experience and phenomena are understood to be dream. This should not be just an intellectual understanding, but a vivid and lucid experience. Otherwise it is just a game of the imagination and no real change is effected. Genuine integration of this point produces a profound change in the individual's response to the world. Grasping and aversion is greatly diminished, and the emotional tangles that once seemed so compelling are experienced as the tug of dream stories, and no more.

As the practice changes the experiences of the visions of the day, the change is integrated into dream. Lucidity arises in the dream state. There are successive levels of lucidity, from the first experiences of being aware that the dream is a dream while still directed by the logic of the dream, to a powerful lucidity in which one is totally free in the dream and dream itself becomes an experience of almost shocking vividness and clarity.

The lucidity and flexibility of mind developed in dream is then to be integrated into the intermediate state after death. Experiencing death is very similar to entering dream. The possibility of remaining present during the intermediate bardo after death, of staying aware and undistracted as the after-death visions arise, depends on the capacities developed in dream yoga. We say that dream is a test for the bardo. This is the integration of the dream state with the intermediate state, understanding that reactions to the phenomena of dream will be the same as reactions to the phenomena of the bardo. The accomplishment at this point depends on the development of lucidity and non-grasping in dream.

The bardo is to be integrated with the clear light. This is the means of achieving enlightenment. During the bardo, it is best not to engage dualistically with the phenomena that arise, but instead remain in nondual presence, in full awareness without distraction. This is remaining in the clear light, the union of emptiness and pure awareness. The ability to do this is also the final stage of dream practice prior to death: when the practitioner fully integrates with the clear light, dreaming stops.

When waking experience is directly seen to be a dream, grasping ceases. The greater lucidity that has to have been developed to progress to this point is naturally brought into the dreams of night. When lucidity is developed and stabilized in dream, it later manifests in the bardo. When one is completely and non-dualistically aware in the bardo, liberation is attained.

Apply dream practice without interruption and the results will manifest in every dimension of life. The result of the full accomplishment of the practice is liberation. If the practice is not resulting in changed experiences of life, if one is not more relaxed with less tension and less distraction, then the obstacles must be investigated and overcome and the teacher should be consulted. If there is no experience of progression on the path, then the intent is best strengthened. When signs of progress do arise, greet them with joy and let them reinforce your intent. With understanding and practice, progress will surely come.

PART FOUR

Sleep

The following sections presuppose some familiarity with basic tantric terminology. Unlike the earlier material on dream yoga, these sections on sleep yoga are primarily addressed to those who are already tantric or Dzogchen practitioners.

1 Sleep and Falling Asleep

The normal process of sleep occurs as consciousness withdraws from the senses and the mind loses itself in distraction, thinning out in mental images and thoughts until it dissolves in darkness. Unconsciousness then lasts until dreams arise. When they do, the sense of self is reconstituted through dualistic relationship with the images of the dream until the next period of unconsciousness occurs. Alternating periods of unconsciousness and dream make up a normal night of sleep.

Sleep is dark to us because we lose consciousness in it. It seems to be empty of experience because we identify with the gross mind, which ceases to function during sleep. The period in which our identities collapse we call "falling asleep." We are conscious in dream because the moving mind is active, giving rise to a dream ego with which we identify. In sleep, however, the subjective self does not arise.

Although we define sleep as unconsciousness, the darkness and experiential blankness are not the essence of sleep. For the pure awareness that is our basis there is no sleep. When not afflicted with obscurations, dreams, or thoughts, the moving mind dissolves into the nature of mind; then, rather than the sleep of ignorance, clarity, peacefulness, and bliss arise. When we develop the ability to abide in that awareness we find that sleep is luminous. This luminosity is the clear light. It is our true nature.

As explained in previous chapters, dreams arise from karmic traces. I used the analogy of light being projected through film to make movies, where the karmic traces are the photographs, awareness is the light that illuminates them, and the dreams are projected on the base (*kunzhi**). Dream yoga develops lucidity in relationship to the dream images. But in sleep yoga there is no film and no projection. Sleep yoga is imageless. The practice is the direct recognition of awareness by awareness, light illuminating itself. It is luminosity without images of any kind. Later, when stability in the clear light is developed, even dream images will not distract the practitioner, and the dream period of sleep will also occur in the clear light. These dreams are then called clear light dreams, which are different than dreams of clarity. In clear light dreams, the clear light is not obscured.

We lose the real sense of the clear light as soon as we conceptualize it or try to imagine it. There is neither subject nor object in the clear light. If there is any identification with a subject, then there is no entry into the clear light. Actually, nothing "enters" the clear light: the clear light is the base recognizing itself. There is neither "you" nor "it." Using dualistic language to describe the non-dual necessarily results in paradox. The only way to know the clear light is to know it directly.

2 Three Kinds of Sleep

SLEEP OF IGNORANCE

The sleep of ignorance, which we call "deep sleep," is a great darkness. It feels like a darkness thousands of years old, and it is even
older: it is the essence of ignorance, the root of samsara. No matter
how many nights we sleep, every night for thirty years or seventy, we
cannot finish sleeping. We return to it again and again as if it recharges
us, and it does. Ignorance is the sustenance of samsara and, as samsaric
beings, when we dissolve into the sleep of ignorance, our samsaric
lives are fed. We wake stronger, our samsaric existence is refreshed.
This is "great ignorance" because it is immeasurable.

We experience the sleep of ignorance as a void or blank, in which
there is no sense of self and no consciousness. Think of a long, tiring
day, rainy weather, a heavy dinner, and the resultant sleep in which
there is neither clarity nor sense of self. We disappear. One manifestation of ignorance in the mind is the mental drowsiness that pulls us
toward such dissolution in unconsciousness.

Innate ignorance is the primary cause of sleep. The necessary secondary causes and conditions for its manifestation are tied to the body
and the body's weariness.

SAMSARIC SLEEP

The second kind of sleep is samsaric sleep, the sleep of dreams.
Samsaric sleep is called "great delusion" because it seems endless.

Samsaric sleep is like going for a walk in the downtown of a big city, where all manner of things take place: people embrace, fight, chat, and abandon one another; there is hunger and wealth; people run businesses and people steal from businesses; there are beautiful places, tattered places, frightening places. Manifestations of the six realms can be found in any city, and samsaric sleep is the city of dreams, a limitless realm of mental activity generated by the karmic traces of past actions. Unlike the sleep of ignorance, in which the gross moving mind ceases, samsaric sleep requires the participation of the gross mind and the negative emotions.

While it is the body that calls us to the sleep of ignorance, emotional activity is the primary cause of dream. The secondary causes are actions based in grasping or aversion.

CLEAR LIGHT SLEEP

The third kind of sleep, which is realized through sleep yoga, is clear light sleep. It is also called the sleep of clarity. It occurs when the body is sleeping but the practitioner is neither lost in darkness nor in dreams, but instead abides in pure awareness.

Clear light is defined in most texts as the unity of emptiness and clarity. It is the pure, empty awareness that is the base of the individual. "Clear" refers to emptiness, the mother, the base, kunzhi. "Light" refers to clarity, the son, rigpa, pure innate awareness. Clear light is direct realization of the unity of rigpa and the base, of awareness and emptiness.

Ignorance is compared to a dark room in which you sleep. Awareness is a lamp in that room. No matter how long the room has been dark, an hour or a million years, the moment the lamp of awareness is lit the entire room becomes luminous. There is a buddha in the flame, the dharmakaya. You are that luminosity. You are the clear light; it is not an object of your experience or a mental state. When the luminous awareness in the darkness is blissful, clear, unmoving, without reference, without judgement, without center or circumference, that is rigpa. It is the nature of mind.

When thought is observed in awareness with neither grasping nor aversion, it dissolves. When the thought—the object of awareness—dissolves, the observer or subject also dissolves. In a sense, when the object dissolves, it dissolves in the base and when the subject dissolves, it dissolves in rigpa. This is a risky example in that one may think there are two things, the base and the rigpa; that would be wrong understanding. They are as inseparable as water and wetness. They are described as two aspects of the same thing to aid us in understanding, to relate the teachings to the apparent dichotomy of subject and object. But the truth is that there is never an object separate from a subject; there is only an illusion of separation.

3 Sleep Practice and Dream Practice

The difference between dream and sleep practice somewhat parallels the difference in the practice of calm abiding (zhine) when an object is used and when there is no object. Similarly, in tantric practice, dream yoga is used to generate the divine body of the meditational deity (yidam), which is still in the realm of subject and object, while sleep yoga develops the mind of the deity, which is pure non-dual awareness. In one sense, dream practice is a secondary practice in Dzogchen because it is still working with vision and images, while in the sleep practice there is neither subject nor object but only non-dual rigpa.

When the student is introduced to Dzogchen practice, practices with attributes are usually taught first. Only after some development of stability is practice without attributes begun. This is because the dominant style of our consciousness has to do with attributes, with objects of the subject with which one is identified. Because we are constantly identified with the activity of the moving mind, in the beginning our practice must provide something for the mind to grasp. If we are told, "Just be space," the moving mind cannot make sense of it, because there is nothing to hold. It tries to make an image of emptiness in order to identify with it, which is not the practice. But if we say that something is to be visualized and then dissolved and so on, the moving mind feels comfortable, because there is something to think. We use the conceptual mind and objects of awareness to lead the mind to awareness without attributes, which is where the practice must go.

For example, we are told to imagine the body dissolving—that sounds fine, it can be pictured. After the dissolution, there is a moment in which there is nothing to grasp, and this provides the situation in which the prepared practitioner can recognize rigpa. It is similar to counting down from ten—ten, nine, eight—until zero is reached. There is nothing to grasp in zero, it is the tigle of empty space, but the movement leads us there. Counting down to emptiness is similar to using practice with attributes to lead us to the emptiness of practice without attributes.

Sleep practice actually has no form, so there is nothing on which to focus. The practice and the goal are the same: to abide in the inseparable unity of clarity and emptiness, beyond dualistic separation of perceiver and perceived. There are no qualities, no up or down, no inside or outside, no top or bottom, no time or boundaries. There are no distinctions at all. Because there is no object for the mind to grasp as there is in dream, sleep yoga is considered more difficult than dream yoga. Becoming lucid in a dream means the dream is recognized; it is the object of awareness. But in sleep practice, the recognition is not of an object by a subject but is the non-dual recognition of pure awareness, the clear light, by awareness itself. The sensory consciousness is not functioning, so the mind that relies on sensory experience is not functioning. The clear light is like seeing without an eye, an object, or a seer.

This is analogous to what occurs in death: it is harder to become liberated in the first bardo, the primordially pure (*ka-dag*) bardo, than in the subsequent bardo, the clear light (*od-sal*) bardo, in which images arise. At the time of death, there is a moment of total dissolution of subjective experience into the base prior to the appearances of the bardo visions. In that moment, there is no subjective self, just as daily experience ends in the dissolution of sleep. We are gone. And then dreams arise in sleep, or images arise in the bardo, and as they are perceived the force of karmic tendencies creates the sense of a perceiving self experiencing the objects of perception. Caught up again in dualism, we continue in samsaric dream if asleep or continue toward rebirth if in the bardo.

If we accomplish sleep practice, we can become liberated in the primordially pure bardo. If we have not accomplished sleep yoga, we will encounter the subsequent bardo visions, during which, if accomplished in dream practice, we are more likely to become liberated. If we have not accomplished either dream or sleep practice, we continue to wander in samsara.

You must decide for yourself which of these practices is most suitable. Dzogchen teachings always stress the importance of knowing yourself, recognizing your capacities and obstacles, and using that knowledge to practice in the manner that will be most beneficial. That said, there are only a few people for whom sleep practice will be easier than dream practice, so I generally recommend beginning with dream practice. If your mind is still grasping, it makes sense to begin with dream yoga, in which the mind can fasten on the dream itself. After stability in rigpa is developed, sleep practice may be easier to accomplish because there is a strong experience of not grasping, of not being a subject, which is the situation in sleep. Another reason I recommend starting with dream yoga is that it usually takes much longer for the practitioner to become lucid in sleep than in dream. Practicing for a long time without apparent results may result in discouragement, which can become an obstruction on the path. Once you have some experience in either of the yogas it is good to continue and reinforce the practice.

The two yogas ultimately lead into one another. When dream practice is fully accomplished, the non-dual awareness of rigpa will manifest in dream. This leads to many dreams of clarity and finally to the dissolution of dreams into the clear light. This is also the fruit of sleep practice. Conversely, when progress is made in sleep yoga, dreams will naturally become lucid and dreams of clarity will spontaneously arise. The lucid dreams can then be used for the development of the flexibility of mind as previously described. Final success in either practice requires that the pure presence of rigpa be recognized and stabilized during the day.

PART FIVE

The Practice of Sleep Yoga

1   The Dakini, Salgye Du Dalma

The *Mother Tantra* teaches that there is a dakini who is the protector and guardian of sacred sleep. It is helpful to make a connection with her essence, which is also the nature of the practice, so that she can guide and bless the transition from unconscious to conscious sleep. Her name is Salgye Du Dalma (*gsal-byed-gdos-bral-ma*). This translates as "She Who Clarifies Beyond Conception." She is the luminosity hidden inside the darkness of normal sleep.

She is formless in sleep practice itself, but as we are falling asleep she is visualized as a luminous sphere of light, a tiglé. Light is visualized, rather than a form like the syllables used in dream yoga, because we are working on the level of energy, beyond form. We are trying to dissolve all distinctions such as inside and outside, self and other. When visualizing a form, it is the habit of the mind to think of that form as something other than itself, and we must go beyond dualism. The dakini is the representation of the clear light. She is what we already are in our pure state: clear and luminous. We become her in sleep practice.

When we develop a relationship with Salgye Du Dalma, we connect to our own deepest nature. We can further this connection by remembering her as much as possible. During the day she can be visualized in *samboghakaya** form: pure white, luminous, and beautiful. Her translucent body is made wholly of light. In her right hand she holds a curved knife, and in her left hand a bowl made from the top of a skull. She abides in the heart center, sitting upon a white moon disc, which rests on a golden sun disk, which in turn rests upon a beautiful blue, four-petaled lotus. As in guru yoga, imagine yourself dissolving into her, and she into you, mixing your essence until it is one.

Wherever you are, she is with you, residing in your heart. When you eat, offer her food. When you drink, offer her what you drink. You can talk to her. If you are in a space in which you can listen, let her talk to you. This does not mean you should go crazy, but you can use your imagination. If you have read books on dharma and listened to talks on these topics, imagine her giving you the teachings that you already know. Let her remind you to remain in presence, to cut through ignorance, to act compassionately, to be mindful, and to resist distractions. Your teacher may not always be available, nor your friends, but the dakini is. Make her your constant companion and the guide of your practice. You will find that eventually the communication will start to feel real; she will embody your own understanding of the dharma and reflect it back to you. When you remember her presence, the room you are in will seem more luminous and your mind will become lucid; she is teaching you that the luminosity and lucidity you experience is the clear light that you really are. Train yourself so that even feelings of disconnection and the arising of negative emotions automatically remind you of her; then confusion and emotional snares will serve to bring you back to awareness like the bell of a temple that marks the beginning of practice.

If this relationship with the dakini sounds too foreign or fanciful, you may wish to psychologize it. That is all right. You can think of her as a separate being or as a symbol that you use to guide your intention and your mind. In either case, devotion and consistency are powerful assets on the spiritual journey. You may also do this practice with your yidam, if you do yidam practice, or with any deity or enlightened being; it is your efforts that make a difference in your practice, not the form. But it is also good to recognize that Salgye Du Dalma is especially associated with this practice in the *Mother Tantra*. There is a long history of practitioners working with her form and her energy, and making a connection with the power of the lineage can be a great support.

Imagination is very powerful, strong enough to bind one to the sufferings of samsara for an entire life, and strong enough to make the dialogue with the dakini real. Often practitioners act toward the dharma as if it is rigid, but it is not. The dharma is flexible and the mind should be flexible with it. It is your responsibility to find how to use the dharma to support your realization. Rather than imagining how the day will go tomorrow, or the fight you had with the boss, or the evening ahead with your partner, it may be more helpful to create the presence of this beautiful dakini who embodies the highest goal of practice. The important point is to develop the powerful intention needed to accomplish the practice and a strong relationship to your true nature, which the dakini represents. As often as possible, pray to her for the sleep of clear light. Your intention will be strengthened each time you do.

Ultimately, you are to become one with the dakini, which does not mean assuming her form as in tantric practice. It means remaining in the nature of mind, being rigpa in every moment. Remaining in the natural state is both the best preliminary and the best practice.

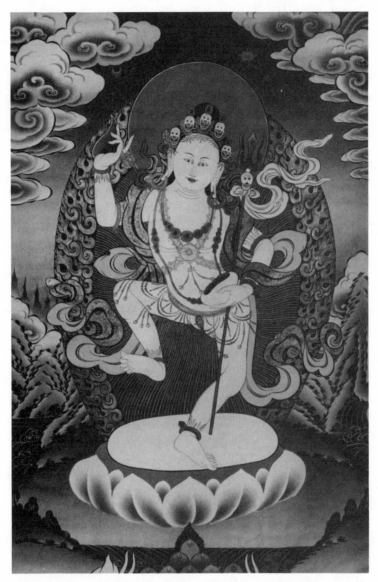

Salgye Du Dalma

2 Preliminary Practice

Stress and tension taken to bed will follow the sleeper into sleep. Therefore, bring the mind into rigpa if possible. If not, then bring the mind into the body, into the central channel, into the heart. The preliminary practices recommended for dream yoga also apply to sleep yoga. Take refuge in the lama, yidam, and dakini, or do the nine breaths of purification and guru yoga. At a minimum, think of good things that promote devotion and practice, such as generating compassion. This anyone can do. Also make prayers for clear light sleep. If you have other practices that you normally do before bed, you may continue doing those.

A candle or small light left on during the night keeps a bit of wakefulness in the mind. It feels different to sleep with a light on, and the difference can be used to help maintain awareness. If a candle is used, be sure to take precautions against fire.

The light not only helps with maintaining alertness, it also represents the dakini, Salgye Du Dalma. The clarity and luminosity of light are closer to her essence than are any other phenomena in the world of form. When a light is on, imagine the luminosity in the room to be the dakini surrounding you with this essence. Let the external light connect you to the internal light, to the luminosity that you are. Relating the experience of light in the physical world to the practice helps; it gives the conventional mind a direction, a support, as it moves toward dissolution in pure awareness. External light can be a bridge between the conceptual world of form and the non-conceptual direct experience of the formless.

Another preliminary practice sometimes used is to go without sleep for one, three, or even five nights. This exhausts the conventional mind. Traditionally, this is done by a practitioner when the teacher is nearby. After the period of sleeplessness, when the practitioner finally sleeps, the master wakes the practitioner periodically during the night and asks questions: Were you aware? Did you dream? Did you fall into the sleep of ignorance?

If you wish to try this, make an arrangement with an experienced practitioner whom you trust. After your sleepless night—it is best to first remain sleepless only for one night—arrange to receive a massage, if possible, to relax the body and open the channels. Then have the practitioner wake you three times during the night and ask the above questions. After each waking, do the practice explained below, and again go to sleep. Sometimes the conventional mind can become so exhausted that it is very quiet. Then it is easier to find oneself in the clear light.

3 Sleep Practice

Four sessions of sleep practice are done during waking periods in the night, as in dream practice. In sleep yoga, however, all four sessions are the same.

Lie in the lion position, as explained in the chapter on dream practice: men on the right side, women on the left. Visualize four blue lotus petals in the heart center. In the center is the dakini, Salgye Du Dalma, visualized in her essence as a luminous, clear sphere of pure light, a tiglé as transparent as perfect crystal. The tiglé, clear and colorless in itself, reflects the blue of the petals and becomes a radiant whitish-blue. Mingle your presence fully with the luminous tiglé to the extent that you become luminous blue light.

On each of the four blue petals is a tiglé, making five with the central tiglé. In front is a yellow tiglé, representing the east. To your left, north, is a green tiglé. Behind is the red tiglé of the west. And to the right is the blue tiglé of the south. The tiglés represent four dakinis visualized in their luminous essence, the colored light. Do not visualize their forms as other than spheres of luminosity. The four tiglés are like a retinue for Salgye Du Dalma. Develop the sense that you are surrounded by the protection of the dakinis; try to really feel this loving presence until you are secure and relaxed.

Pray to the dakini that you have the sleep of clear light rather than dreams or the sleep of ignorance. Make your prayer strong and devoted, and pray again and again. Prayer will help to strengthen devotion and intention. It cannot be overemphasized that strong intention is the foundation of the practice. Developing devotion will aid in making intention one-pointed and powerful enough to pierce the clouds of ignorance that mask the luminosity of the clear light.

ENTERING SLEEP

Although the experience of falling asleep is continuous, it is divided into five stages as an aid in bringing awareness to the process. In the table below, the column on the left lists a progressive disconnection from the senses and sense objects until there is a total "absence of vision," which means a complete lack of sensory experience.

Normally, identity is dependent on the world of the senses. As that world disappears in sleep, the support for consciousness collapses and the result is "falling asleep," which means we become unconscious. Sleep yoga uses the tiglés to support consciousness as contact with the external world is lost. Corresponding with the progressive dissolution of sensory experience, the practitioner connects, in sequence, to the five tiglés, until, with the external world completely gone, the subject dissolves in the pure non-dual luminosity of the clear light. The movement from one tiglé to another should be as smooth as possible in keeping with the continuous and unsegmented movement toward sleep.

a. After you lie down in the proper position, sensory experience remains full: you see through your eyes, you hear, you feel the bed, and so on. This is the moment of vision. The conventional self is supported by sensory experience. Begin to shift that support to the pure

STAGES IN CESSATION OF SENSORY ENGAGEMENT			
Sensory Experience	**Tiglé**		
	Color	Direction	Location
a. Vision	Yellow	East	Front
b. Vision decreasing	Green	North	Left
c. Vision declining	Red	West	Rear
d. Vision ceasing	Blue	South	Right
e. Vision absent	Whitish-Blue	Center	Center

consciousness that the tiglés represent. The first step is to merge your awareness with the tiglé to the front, a beautiful, warm yellow light in which the conceptual mind can begin to dissolve.

b. When the eyes close, contact with the sensory world begins to diminish. This is the second point, in which vision decreases. As external support is lost, shift awareness to the green tiglé on the left. Allow identity to begin to dissolve as sense experience diminishes.

c. As sensory experience becomes more muted, shift awareness to the red tiglé. The process of going to sleep is familiar—the softening and blurring of the senses, the gradual loss of sensation. Normally, as the external supports of identity are lost, you lose yourself, but now you are learning to exist without any support.

d. When sensory experience is almost extinguished, move the awareness into the blue tiglé on the right. This is the period when all sensory experience ceases. It is very quiet in all the senses and there is barely any contact with the external world.

e. Finally, as the body completely enters sleep and all contact with the body's senses is lost, awareness fully merges with the central whitish-blue tiglé. By this point, if you are successful, the tiglé will not actually be an object of awareness; you will not visualize a blue light nor will you define experience by location. Rather, you will be the clear light itself; you are to abide in this during sleep.

Notice that these five stages do not refer to inner, mental appearances, but to the gradual cessation of sensory experience. Ordinarily, the sleeper moves through this process unconsciously; with this practice the process is to take place in awareness. The steps in the process should not be clearly demarcated. As consciousness withdraws from the senses, allow the awareness to move smoothly through the tiglés until only non-dual awareness—the clear light of the central tiglé— remains. It is as if the body spirals down into sleep while you spiral down into the clear light. Rather than relying on conceptual decisions to move from one tiglé to the next, and rather than trying to make the process happen, allow intention to unfold the process in experience.

If you wake fully in the middle of the practice, start again. You need not be too rigid with the form of the practice. Nor does it matter whether the process occurs quickly or slowly. For some people, falling asleep is drawn out; others fall asleep seconds after their head touches the pillow. Both go through the same transition. A needle passes almost instantly through a pile of five gossamer wings but there are still five moments in which it goes through each wing in turn. Do not be too analytical about which stage is which or get caught up in dividing the process neatly into five. The visualization is only a support for awareness in the beginning. The essence of the practice must be understood and applied rather than lost in the details.

In my own experience, I have found the practice is also effective when the tiglés are engaged in the opposite direction. Then, you visualize the yellow tiglé in front, representing earth; the blue tiglé to the right, representing water; the red tiglé to the rear, representing fire; the green tiglé to the left, representing air; and finally the whitish-blue tiglé in the center, representing space. This sequence parallels the sequence in which the elements dissolve in death. You can experiment to determine which sequence works best for you.

As in dream practice, it is best to wake three times during the night, spaced in roughly two-hour intervals. Once experience is developed, you can use the natural moments of waking in the night rather than three scheduled waking periods. Repeat the same practice in each period of waking. Each time you awake, examine the experience of the sleep from which you have just awoken: Did you lack all awareness and thus sleep the sleep of ignorance? Did you dream, lost in samsaric sleep? Or were you in the clear light, abiding in pure nondual awareness?

4 Tiglé

Tiglé has many different definitions, each appropriate in different contexts. In the context of this practice it is a small sphere of light representing particular qualities of consciousness or, in the case of the central tiglé, representing pure rigpa. Although ultimately awareness must be stable without relying on any object, until that capacity is developed light is a useful support. Light is luminous and clear, and although it is still in the world of form, it is less substantial than any other perceptible form. The visualization of the tiglés is a bridge, a crutch useful until even perceptible light can be abandoned and the practitioner can abide in imageless, empty, awareness, in the luminosity that is the essence of light.

When the tiglé is visualized on the four blue petals in the heart chakra, it is not necessary to try to determine the exact anatomical site. What is important is to sense the center of the body in the area of the heart. Use awareness and imagination to find the right place, the place in which there is actual experience.

The colors of the tiglés are not chosen at random. Color affects the quality of consciousness, and the colored lights are meant to evoke particular qualities that are to be integrated in the practice, much as the specific chakras, colors, and syllables form a progression in dream yoga. The different qualities can be experienced as we move from one tiglé to the other—yellow, green, red, blue—to the extent that we allow ourselves to be sensitive to the differences.

This is not a transformation practice, in which we would transform our identity; in sleep yoga, identity is given up altogether. It is not the point to stay with a visualization, as it might be in a tantric practice. But the mind must have something to hold; if it does not have the light, it will grab something else.

Before we have experience of rigpa, it is difficult to imagine how we can remain aware with neither a subject nor an object of awareness. Normally, consciousness requires an object, which is what is meant by consciousness being "supported" by a form or attribute. The practices in which the visualized object or the subjective identity is dissolved train the practitioner to remain aware as dualistic supports for consciousness disappear. They prepare us for sleep yoga, but they are not like sleep yoga itself. Even "practice" is a support, and in actual sleep yoga there is no support and no practice: the yoga is accomplished or it is not, as the mind that relies on support dissolves into the base.

5 Progress

Usually when one drives along a familiar route, awareness of the present is lost. Even during a daily commute lasting forty-five minutes or an hour, nothing is really seen with strong awareness. The driver is on automatic, lost in thoughts about the job or fantasies about a vacation or worry about the bills or plans for the family.

Then one becomes a practitioner and decides to remain as present as possible during the drive home, to use the time as an opportunity to strengthen the mind for practice. It is very difficult to do, because of conditioning. The mind repeatedly floats away. The practitioner brings it back—to the feel of the steering wheel, the color of the grass along the highway—but this only lasts for a minute before the mind's activity carries the attention away again.

It is the same with meditation practice. The mind is placed on the image of a deity, or on *A*, or on the breath; a minute later it wanders off again. It may take a long time, even years, before presence can be maintained continuously for a half hour.

When dream practice is begun, it follows a similar progression. Most dreams are periods of complete distraction; the dream is forgotten almost as quickly as it happens. With practice, moments of lucidity arise, gradually increasing to long minutes of lucid presence in dream. Even then, the lucidity may be lost, or the next dream may again be lacking lucidity. Progress is made, it is certain and recognizable, but it takes diligence and strong intention.

Sleep practice is often even slower to develop. But if, after a long time of practice, there is no progress—no increased presence, no recognizable positive changes in life—it is best not to accept this state of affairs. Rather, do purification practices, examine and heal broken commitments (samaya), or work with the prana and energy of the body. Other practices may be needed to clear obstacles and serve as a basis for the accomplishment of dream and sleep yogas.

The practitioner is like a vine that can only grow where there is support. External circumstances have a strong influence on the quality of life, so try to spend time in environments and with people that support practice rather than detract from it. It helps to read books on the dharma, practice meditation with others, attend teachings, and to associate with other practitioners. Practitioners have the responsibility to honestly evaluate their practice and its results. If this is not done, it is easy to spend many years believing progress is being made when nothing is actually happening.

6 Obstacles

Sleep yoga is not only a practice for sleep. It is the practice of remaining in non-dual awareness continually, throughout the four states of waking, sleeping, meditation, and death. Thus, the obstacles addressed below are actually the single obstacle of being driven away from the clear light and into dualistic, samsaric experience. The obstacles are:

1. Losing the presence of the natural clear light of day when distracted by sensory or mental phenomena

2. Losing the presence of the clear light of sleep when distracted by dreams

3. Losing the presence of the clear light of samadhi (during meditation) when distracted by thought

4. Losing the presence of the clear light of death when distracted by the visions of the intermediate state

1. Losing the presence of the natural clear light of day. The obstacle during waking life is external appearance. We become lost in the experiences, the visions, of the sense objects. A sound comes and takes us away, a smell comes and we are lost in a daydream of fresh-baked bread, the wind tickles the hair on the neck and we lose the center-less awareness of rigpa and instead become a subject experiencing the sensation. If we remain in the clarity of rigpa, experience is different. A sound arises but we are connected to the silence in it and do not lose presence. A vision passes before us but we are rooted in stillness and remain in the unmoving mind. The way to overcome the obstacle of external appearance is to develop stability in the natural clear light.

The natural clear light is the clear light of the day, the same as the clear light of the night. Knowing the clear light of the day we can also find the clear light during sleep. The practice is to connect the natural clear light of waking life to the clear light of sleep and the clear light of samadhi, until we continuously abide in pure rigpa.

2. *Losing the presence of the clear light of sleep.* The obstacle to realizing the clear light of sleep is dream. When a dream arises, we react to it dualistically and engage in the fiction of being a subject in a world of objects. This is similar to the first obstacle, but is now internal rather than external. We say images obscure the clear light; however, it is not that the dream actually obscures clarity, but that we are distracted from clarity. This is why, in the beginning of practice, we pray to have neither the sleep of ignorance nor the sleep of dream. When enough stability is developed, dream no longer distracts us and the result is the clear light dream.

3. *Losing the presence of the clear light of samadhi.* The clear light of samadhi is the meditative clear light or consciousness clear light. This is rigpa during meditation practice. Thoughts are the obscuration of the clear light of samadhi in the early stages of practice. When stability is developed in rigpa during practice, then we can learn to integrate thought with rigpa. Until then, when a thought arises we grasp at it or push it away and are distracted from rigpa.

This should not be taken as an indication that the meditative clear light is only found after many years of practice. There are many moments of life in which the natural clear light can be found; in fact it can be found at any moment. The key is whether or not you are introduced to it and can recognize it.

4. *Losing the presence of the clear light of death.* The clear light of death is obscured by the bardo visions. The clarity of rigpa is lost when we are distracted by the visions that arise after death and enter into dualistic relationship with them. As with the other three obstacles, this loss does not have to occur if there is sufficient stability in the clear light.

The bardo need not obscure the clear light of death. Thoughts need not obscure the samadhi clear light. Dream need not obscure the clear light of sleep. External objects need not obscure the natural clear light.

If we are deluded by these four obstacles, we will not pass from samsara; there is only the falling back into samsaric traps. Having accomplished sleep and dream practices, we will know how to transform these obscurations into the path.

Sleep practice is not just for sleep, but is the practice of integrating all moments—waking and sleeping, dreaming and in the bardo—with the clear light. When this is done, liberation is the result. Mystical experiences and insights, as well as all thoughts, feelings, and perceptions, can arise within the presence of rigpa. When they do, allow them to spontaneously self-liberate, dissolving in emptiness, leaving no karmic trace. All experience is then direct, immediate, vivid, and fulfilling.

7 Supportive Practices

Below are short descriptions of practices, most of them recommendations from the Mother Tantra, *that are supportive of the main sleep practice.*

MASTER

To support the sleep practice, generate stronger devotion to one's true nature. Imagine the master at the crown of the head and develop connection and devotion. The connection to the master can be very pure, based in pure devotion. When you imagine the master, go beyond just visualizing an image: generate strong devotion and really feel the presence of the master. Pray with strength and sincerity. Then dissolve the master into light that enters your crown and descends into your heart. Imagine the master abiding there, in your heart center, then go to sleep.

The closeness that you feel to the master is actually the closeness you feel toward your own nature. This is the support of the lama.

DAKINI

On a radiant lotus in the heart, seated on a sun disk that sits on the lotus, abides the dakini Salgye Du Dalma. She is clear, translucent, and luminous, like a bright light. Feel her presence strongly, feel her compassion and care. She is protecting you, aiding you, leading you. She is the ally that you can whole-heartedly depend upon. She is the essence of the clear light, your goal, enlightenment. Generate love for her, and trust and respect. She is the illumination that comes with realization. Focusing on her and praying to her, fall asleep.

BEHAVIOR

Go to a quiet place where there are no other people. Cover your body with ashes. Eat heavier foods that help to overcome wind disorders. Then jump wildly around, fully expressing whatever is inside, letting out whatever blocks or distracts you. No one is around, so explode if need be. Let this catharsis clean you and relax you. Act out all your tensions. With great fervor pray to the master, the yidam, the dakini, and the refuge tree; pray strongly, asking for the experience of clear light. Then sleep inside of that awakening experience.

PRAYER

If you have not had the experiences of the clear light of day, meditation, and sleep, pray for these results again and again. It is easy to forget about the simple power of wish and prayer. We think that prayer must be something extraordinary, directed to some incredible power external to us, but this is not the case. The important point is to feel strongly the intent and desire in the prayer, to put our heart in it.

Originally, perhaps, when people wished one another good night or good morning, or to sleep well, there was some power in the words, some feeling. Now these are just habitual phrases that we mutter mechanically, with little feeling or meaning. The same words are used, they are spoken in the same tone, but they are without power. Be careful not to do this with prayer. Know that prayer has power but it is not in the words; it is in the feeling you put in the prayer. Develop intention, make it strong, and put it into the prayer.

DISSOLVING

Doing this exercise can give a sense of how the focusing in the practice should be. The practice begins with light and the perceiver of light, but the intent is to unify the two.

Relax fully. Shut your eyes and begin with a precise visualization of the whitish-blue tiglé, about the size of a thumbprint, in the heart center. Slowly let it expand and grow more diffuse. It is good to see the light of the tiglé but more important to feel it. Let the light radiate from your heart. As the beautiful blue light shines out, it dissolves everything it touches. Dissolve the room you are in, the house, the town, the state, the country. Dissolve every part of the world, the solar system, the entire universe. Every point the mind touches—whether place, person, thing, thought, image, or feeling—dissolve. The three worlds of desire, form, and the formless—dissolve. When everything external is dissolved into light, then let the light come to you. Let it dissolve your body, so that your body turns into blue light and merges with the blue light around it. Then dissolve your mind—every thought, every mental event. Dissolve all the problems in your life. Merge with the light. Become the light. Now there is no inner or outer, no you or not you. There is no sense of a substantial world or self. There is only the luminosity in the space of the heart, which is now pervasive space. Experience still arises, but allow whatever arises to dissolve spontaneously in blue light. Let this happen without effort. There is only light. Then slowly dissolve even the light into space.

It is here you should remain during sleep.

EXPANDING AND CONTRACTING

This is a similar but more formal practice meant to support sleep yoga. Visualize thousands of blue *HUNGs* coming from both nostrils with the exhalation. They originate in the heart and travel up the channels to leave the nostrils with the breath. As they spread out, pervading all space and all dimensions, they dissolve everything they encounter. Their luminosity illuminates all space. With the inhalation, the light of the *HUNGs* returns, illuminating and dissolving body and mind, until there is no inner or outer. Do this visualization until there is only the expanding and contracting light of the *HUNGs*. Dissolve into this light, and abide in the non-dual state. Do this for twenty-one breaths, or more if you can. Practice this during the day as often as possible.

The mind plays tricks. Its main trick is to identify itself as the subject and then take everything else to be separate from that subject. In this practice, everything perceived as outside of yourself is dissolved on the exhalation. The perceiver is dissolved on the inhalation. Both outside and inside become luminous and clear and merge into one

The Tibetan Syllable HUNG

another, becoming indistinguishable. Whenever the mind finds a door to escape into distraction, let awareness follow after it with blue *HUNG*s. When the mind reaches for an object, dissolve the object in light. When the mind returns and fixes on itself as a subject, then dissolve that, too. Eventually, even the sense of solidity can dissolve, the sense of here and there, of objects and subjects, of things and entities.

Generally we think of doing this kind of practice as an aid in generating clear light experience, but it is also helpful in prolonging the experience once it is known and in supporting the continuity of experience.

8 Integration

Once rigpa is known, all of life is to be integrated with it. This is the function of practice. Life needs to take some form; if we do not shape it, it will take a form dictated by karma, which we may not like very much. As the practice is increasingly integrated with life, many positive changes will occur.

INTEGRATION OF CLEAR LIGHT WITH THE THREE POISONS

The clear light must be integrated with the three root poisons: ignorance, desire, and hatred.

Sleep yoga is used to integrate the first, ignorance, with the clear light.

Integrating desire into clear light is similar to discovering the clear light in sleep. When we are lost in the darkness of sleep, the clear light is hidden from us. When we are lost in desire, too, our true nature is obscured, but whereas the sleep of ignorance obscures everything completely, even the sense of self, desire obscures rigpa in particular situations. It makes for a strong separation between the subject and the object of desire. The "wanting" itself is a constriction of consciousness arising from the feeling of lack that remains as long as we do not abide in our true nature. Although the purest desire is the longing for the wholeness and completion of full realization of rigpa, because we do not directly know the nature of mind, the desire becomes attached to other things.

If we directly observe desire rather than becoming fixated on the object of desire, the desire dissolves. And if we can abide in pure presence, the desire, the desiring subject, and the object of desire will all dissolve into their empty essence, revealing the clear light.

We can also use the satisfaction of desire as a means of practice. There is joy in the union of emptiness and clarity. In Tibetan iconography, this is represented in the *yab yum* figures, the forms of male and female deities in union. These forms represent the non-dual unity of wisdom and method, emptiness and clarity, kunzhi and rigpa. The joy of union is present in any unification of apparent dualities, including the desiring subject and the desired object. At the moment when a desire is satisfied, the desire ceases and the apparent duality between desiring subject and object of desire collapses. When that duality collapses, the base, the kunzhi, is there, exposed, though the force of our karmic habits usually carries us into the next movement of duality, leaving a gap in our experience, almost an unconsciousness, rather than the experience of rigpa.

For example, there is the practice of sexual union between man and woman. Normally our experience of orgasm is one of pleasant dreaminess, almost unconsciousness, an exhaustion of desire and restlessness that comes about through fulfillment of desire. But we can integrate that bliss with awareness; rather than becoming lost, if we maintain full awareness without separating the experience into an observing subject and the experience being observed, we can use the situation to find the sacred. The moving mind drops away for a moment and reveals the empty base; integrating that moment with awareness, we have the integration of emptiness and bliss that is spoken of particularly in tantric teachings.

There are many such situations in which we normally lose ourselves and which can instead be moments in which we find our true nature. We do not become lost only in orgasm or intense pleasure. Even in small pleasures we generally lose presence and become bound in the feelings or objects of pleasure. Instead, we can train ourselves so that pleasure itself is a reminder to come to full awareness, to bring awareness to the present moment, the body, the senses, and to let go of distraction. This is one way to integrate desire with clear light. And it is not limited to any particular category of experience; it can be done in any dualistic situation in which there is subject and object. When pleasure is used as a door to practice, the pleasure is not lost; we need not be anti-pleasure. When the subject and object dissolve in clear light, then the union of emptiness and clarity is experienced and there is joy.

The approach to hatred or aversion is similar. If we observe anger rather than participating in it or identifying with it or being driven by it, then the dualistic obsession with the object of anger ceases and the anger dissolves into emptiness. If presence is maintained in that emptiness, then the subject, too, dissolves. The presence in that empty space is the clear light.

By "observing in pure presence" it is not meant that we remain as an angry self, observing the anger, but that we are rigpa, the space in which the anger is occurring. When observed in this way, the anger dissolves into empty essence. Where it dissolves is space. That is the clear. But still there is awareness, presence. That is the light. That emptiness and presence are integrated with anger because anger is no longer obscuring the clear light. If we observe thoughts this way, and if observer and observed both disappear, then there is some experience of rigpa.

Dzogchen is not complicated. The Dzogchen texts often have such lines as, "I am so simple that you cannot understand me. I am so close to you that you cannot see me." When we look far away, we lose awareness of what is close to us. When we look to the future, we lose the present. This happens in every dimension of experience.

Tibetans have a saying: "The more wisdom is present, the less thoughts there will be." It suggests a two-way process. As practice becomes clear and stable, thoughts will dominate experience less. Some people are afraid of this, afraid that if they let go of anger, for example, they will not address what is wrong in the world, as if they need anger to motivate them. But this need not be true. As practitioners, it is important to be responsible for our conventional lives. When bad things happen, they must be taken care of; when something is wrong, it must be addressed. But if we do not see something wrong, we need not go looking for it. Instead, remain in the natural state. If we have anger, we must work with it. But if we do not have anger, we are not missing anything of importance.

I meet many people who say they are Dzogchenpas, practitioners of Dzogchen, and are integrated. There is another Tibetan saying: "When I go up to the steep and difficult places in the borderlands between Tibet and Nepal, I pray to the Three Jewels. When I come down to the beautiful flowery valley, I sing songs." It is easy to say we are integrated when things are easy. But when a strong emotional crisis comes it is the real test; are we Dzogchenpas or not? There is a precision in the practice of Dzogchen. We can discover for ourselves how integrated we are with the practice just by paying attention to how we react to the situations that arise in our lives. When a partner leaves, the partner we dearly love, then where do the beautiful words of integration go? We experience pain; and even this must be integrated.

INTEGRATION WITH THE CYCLES OF TIME

Traditionally, a practice is discussed in terms of view, meditation, and behavior. This section is about behavior. Behavior is described relative to external, internal, and secret unifications with periods of time.

Generally we lose energy and presence as we move through the day. Instead, in developing the practice, we learn to use the passage of time to move us toward a more stable experience of the clear light.

External Unification: Integrating the Clear Light into the Cycle of Day and Night

For the purposes of the practice, the twenty-four hour cycle of day and night is divided into periods that can then be used as supports in developing continuity in the clear light of pure presence. People in the past followed schedules set by the natural cycle of day and night, but this is no longer true. If your schedule is different—perhaps, for example, you work at night—then adapt the teachings to your situation. Although the time of day does affect us energetically, we need not believe that the position of the sun determines the experiences that the teachings describe. Instead, think about these times of day as metaphors for internal processes. The *Mother Tantra* labels the four periods as follows:

1. Dissolution of phenomena in the base
2. Consciousness reaching nirvana
3. Arising of innate awareness to consciousness
4. Equalizing the two truths during the waking state

1. Dissolution of phenomena in the base. The first period is considered to be the time between sunset and going to bed, the evening. During this period, everything seems to be growing dark. Sensory objects become unclear and sensory experience is reduced. The internal sense organs diminish in power. The *Mother Tantra* uses the metaphor of many small rivers moving toward the sea: external phenomena, the senses, the conventional self, thoughts, emotions, and consciousness are moving toward dissolution in sleep, in the base.

You can use imagination to experience this process during the evening. Rather than going toward darkness, move toward the greater light of your true nature. Rather than being fragmented, spread out in the rivers and tributaries of experience, flow toward the wholeness of rigpa. Normally we are connected to the rivers, which are emptying, but the practice is to remain connected to the sea, the base, which is filling. Everything is moving toward the vast, peaceful, radiant sea of the clear light. As night approaches, flow toward completion in non-dual awareness rather than toward unconsciousness.

This is the first of the four periods.

2. Consciousness reaching nirvana. The second period begins when you fall asleep and ends when you wake in the morning, traditionally at dawn. Imagine that period, the quietness of it, the stillness. The text says that when everything becomes dark, a light arises. This is similar to a dark retreat, which is very dark when you enter but soon fills with light.

Try to remain in presence during sleep, fully integrated with the clear light. After external appearances, thought, and feeling dissolve into the base, if you remain in presence it is almost like entering *nirvana*, in which all samsaric experience ceases. It is completely empty, yet there is bliss. When this is realized, it is the union of bliss and emptiness. This is seeing the light in the darkness.

It is not that you should wait until sleep to have clear light experience. Try to abide in the clear light even before falling asleep. Even while working with the visualizations of sleep yoga, remain in rigpa, if possible.

This is the second period, in which the senses and consciousness are like a mandala of the clear sky. Contemplate in that state as much as possible until morning.

3. Arising of innate awareness to consciousness. The third period starts when you wake from sleep and continues until the mind is fully active. The text says that this period lasts from dawn until the sun comes out.

Imagine the quality of that time: the first glimmers of light appear in the dark sky and expand into the beauty of the day. The quiet fills with the sounds of activity, of birds or traffic or people. Internally, it is the movement from the quiet of sleep to full engagement with daily life.

The teachings recommend arising very early in the morning. Wake, if possible, in the nature of mind rather than in the conventional mind. Observe without identifying with the observer. This can be a little easier in the first moments of waking because the conceptual mind is not totally awake yet. Develop the intention to wake in pure presence.

4. *Equalizing the two truths during the waking state.* The fourth period begins when you are fully engaged with the day and ends with sunset. This is day, the time of activity, being busy, and relating to other people. It is full immersion in the world, in forms, language, feelings, smells, and so on. The senses are completely active and occupied with their objects. Still, you should try to continue in the pure presence of rigpa.

Losing yourself in experience, you are confounded by the world. But abiding in the nature of mind, you will find no question to be asked or answered. Being in profound non-dual presence satisfies all questions. Knowing this one thing cuts all doubt.

This is the fourth period, in which conventional and ultimate truth are equalized in the unity of clarity and emptiness.

Internal Unification: Integrating the Clear Light into the Sleep Cycle
The progression described in this section is similar to that in the previous section. Rather than addressing the twenty-four-hour cycle, however, it focuses on developing continuity of presence during the cycle of one waking and one sleeping period, whether it be a nap or an entire night. Before going to sleep, we have to remember that we have the opportunity to practice. This is something positive, something we can do for both practice and health. If the practice feels like a burden, it is better not to do it until inspiration and joyful effort are developed.

Again, there are four periods:
1. Before falling asleep
2. After falling asleep
3. After waking and before becoming fully engaged in the activities of the world
4. The period of activity until the next period of sleep

1. *Before falling asleep.* This spans the time from the moment of lying down until sleep comes. All experience is dissolving into the base; the rivers flow into the sea.

2. *After falling asleep.* The *Mother Tantra* compares this to the dharmakaya, the clear light. The external world of the senses is void yet awareness remains.

3. *After waking.* The clarity is there, the grasping mind is not yet awake. This is like the perfected samboghakaya, not only void but with total clarity.

4. *The period of activity.* When the grasping mind becomes active, that very moment is similar to the manifestation of the nirmanakaya. Activities, thoughts, and the conventional world "start," yet clear light is retained. The world of experience manifests in the non-duality of rigpa.

Secret Unification: Integrating the Clear Light with the Bardo
This practice has to do with integrating the clear light with the intermediate state after death, the bardo. The process of death parallels the process of falling asleep. It is here divided into four stages similar to those of the preceding sections.

1. Dissolution
2. Arising
3. Experiencing
4. Integrating

1. *Dissolution.* In the first stage of death, as the elements of the body begin to disintegrate, sensory experience dissolves, the energies of the internal elements are released, the emotions cease, the life force dissolves, and consciousness dissolves.

2. *Arising.* This is the first bardo after death, the primordially pure (*ka-dag*) bardo. This is like the moment of falling asleep, ordinarily a period of unconsciousness. The accomplished yogi can release all dualistic identities and become liberated directly into the clear light at this stage.

3. *Experiencing.* The bardo of visionary experience arises, the clear light (*od-sal*) bardo. This is similar to arising from the blankness of sleep into a dream, when consciousness is manifest in various forms. Most people will identify with one part of the experience, constituting a

dualistic self, and react dualistically to the apparent objects of consciousness, just as in a samsaric dream. In this bardo, also, the prepared and accomplished yogi can attain liberation.

4. *Integrating.* Next is the bardo of existence (*si-pé-bar-do*). The prepared practitioner unifies conventional reality with non-dual rigpa. This is again the equalization of the two truths, conventional and absolute. If this capacity has not been developed, the individual identifies with the delusory conventional self and relates dualistically to the projections of mind that make up the visionary experience. Rebirth in one of the six realms is the result.

These four periods are stages in the process of dying. We must be aware in them in order to connect to the clear light. When approaching death, we should, if possible, abide in rigpa before sensory experience begins to dissolve. Do not wait until entering the bardo. When hearing has gone but vision remains, for example, it is a signal to be completely present rather than to be distracted by the other senses. Completely let go into rigpa; this is the best preparation for what is to come.

All the dream and sleep practices are, on one level, preparations for death. Death is a crossroads: everyone who dies goes one way or the other. What happens depends on the stability of the practice, whether or not one is able to abide fully in rigpa. Even in a sudden death such as happens in a car crash, there is always a moment in which to recognize—even though it may be harder to do so—that death has come. Right after that recognition, one must try to integrate with the nature of mind.

Many people have had near-death experiences. They say that afterwards the fear of death is gone. This is because they have lived that moment, they know it. When we think about the moment of death, we are not living the reality but are in a fantasy of it that contains more fear than does the actual moment. When the fear goes, integrating with the practice becomes easier.

The Three Unifications: Conclusion

All three of these situations—the cycle of the twenty-four-hour day, the cycle of sleeping and waking, and the process of death—follow a similar sequence. First there is dissolution; then the dharmakaya, emptiness; then the samboghakaya, clarity; then the nirmanakaya, manifestation. The principle is always to remain in non-dual presence.

The division of processes—as in the dream and sleep yogas—is simply to make it easier to bring our awareness into the passing moments, to give us something to look toward, to train us to use inevitable experiences as a support for the practice of pure presence.

Behavior is related to the external process of time. There is no break to the natural state of mind unless we break from it. To connect all experience to the practice, be aware. Of course, secondary circumstances can be helpful for practice; that is why time is introduced as a secondary circumstance. The early morning is helpful, or the day after not sleeping, or when we are exhausted, or when we are completely at rest. There are many moments conducive to integration, such as the moment of release we feel when we really need to go to the toilet and go, or the experience of orgasm, or when we are completely exhausted from carrying something heavy and then put it down and rest. Even every exhalation of breath is a support for the experience of rigpa, if done with awareness. There are many moments when we are partially exhausted and partially awake. We have to bring ourselves to that which is always awake; then we can wake up what is exhausted and sleeping. When we are identified with what grows tired and falls asleep, wakefulness is obscured. But clouds never truly obscure the light of the sun, only the one who is perceiving the sun.

9 Continuity

Because we habitually identify with the fabrications of the mind, we do not find the clear light during sleep. For the same reason, our waking life is distracted, dreamy, and unclear. Rather than experiencing pristine, non-dual rigpa, we remain trapped in the experiences of fantasy and mental projections.

Yet awareness is continuous. Even when asleep, if someone softly says our name, we hear and respond. And during the day, even when most distracted, we remain aware of our environment; we do not simply fall down insensate or walk into walls. In this sense, there is always presence, but the awareness, though unceasing, is foggy and obscured. Piercing the obscurations of ignorance at night, we enter and abide in the radiant clear light. And if we pierce the delusions and hazy fantasies of the moving mind during waking life, we find the same underlying pure awareness of buddha-nature. The distraction of our daily life and the unconsciousness of sleep are two faces of the same ignorance.

The only limits to practice are those we create. It is best not to compartmentalize practice into periods of meditating, dreaming, sleeping, and so on. Ultimately we must abide in rigpa completely in all moments, waking and sleeping. Until then, the practice should be applied in every moment. It is not that we must do every practice we learn. Experiment with the practices, try to understand what the essence and method of the practices are, then discover which practices actually further development and do those until stability in rigpa is attained. The components of the practice are provisional. The position of the body, the preparations, the visualizations, even sleep itself, are not important once one directly knows and abides in the clear light. The experience of clear light is reached through the particulars of the practice, but once it is reached there is no need for practice. There is only clear light.

PART SIX

Elaborations

What follows is additional commentary, relevant to both dream and sleep yogas, to help ground the practice in understanding.

1 Context

In tantra and Dzogchen, the connection between the student and the teacher is extremely important. The student must receive transmission and instruction from the teacher and then must develop some stability in rigpa. Without this, distinctions fundamental to the spiritual journey are difficult to understand because they remain conceptual discriminations. The nature of mind is beyond concepts. Without intellectual understanding it is difficult to develop experience, but without experience the teachings may become, for the practitioner, only abstract philosophy or dogma. It would be like learning about medicine but not recognizing one's own illness; if the knowledge is not used, it is useless. It does no good to merely think that one is in rigpa or to think that one knows the clear light. Knowing and remaining in the view is not merely thinking and talking about the teachings, but actually living in the experience to which the teachings point. The practitioner learns what rigpa is by being rigpa, and discovers the wisdom beyond the conceptual mind by discovering that one's true nature is that wisdom.

Nevertheless, a correct intellectual understanding of the context of dream and sleep yogas helps the practitioner stay directed in practice, avoid error, and prepare to recognize the fruit of the practice. With a clear understanding, the practitioner can check his or her experience against the teaching and avoid the error of mistaking some other experience for rigpa. But finally, these experiences should be checked against the oral teachings given by a teacher during the course of an ongoing relationship, however infrequent the meetings between teacher and student may be.

2 Mind and Rigpa

Liberation from ignorance and suffering occurs when we recognize and abide in our true nature. That which recognizes is not the conceptual mind; it is the fundamental mind, the nature of mind, rigpa. Our necessary task is to distinguish, in practice, between the conceptual mind and the pure awareness of the nature of mind.

CONCEPTUAL MIND

The conceptual or moving mind is the familiar mind of everyday experience, constantly busy with thoughts, memories, images, internal dialogues, judgements, meanings, emotions, and fantasies. It is the mind normally identified as "me" and "my experience." Its fundamental dynamic is engagement with a dualistic vision of existence. It takes itself to be a subject in a world of objects. It grasps at some parts of experience and pushes others away. It is reactive, wildly so sometimes, but even when it is extremely calm and subtle—for example, during meditation or intense concentration—it maintains the internal posture of an entity observing its environment and continues to participate in dualism.

The conceptual mind is not limited to language and ideas. Language—with its nouns and verbs, subjects and objects—is necessarily subject to dualism, but the conceptual mind is active in us before the acquisition of language. Animals have a conceptual mind, in this sense, as do infants and those born without the capacity for language. It is the result of habitual karmic tendencies that are present before we develop a sense of self, even before we are born. Its essential characteristic is that it instinctively divides experience dualistically, beginning with subject and object, with me and not-me.

The *Mother Tantra* refers to this mind as the "active manifestation mind." It is the mind that arises dependent on the movement of karmic prana, and manifests in form as thoughts, concepts, and other mental activities. If the conceptual mind becomes completely still, it dissolves into the nature of mind and will not arise again until activity reconstitutes it.

The moving mind's activities are virtuous, non-virtuous, or neutral. Virtuous actions host the experience of the nature of mind. Neutral actions disturb the connection to the nature of mind. Non-virtuous actions create more disturbance and lead to further disconnection. The teachings go into detail regarding the discriminations between virtuous and non-virtuous actions, such as generosity and greediness and so on. This, however, is the clearest distinction: some actions lead to greater connection to rigpa and some lead to disconnection.

The ego bound by the duality of subject and object arises from the moving mind. From this mind all suffering arises; the conceptual mind works very hard, and this is what it accomplishes. We live in memories of the past and fantasies of the future, cut off from the direct experience of the radiance and beauty of life.

NON-DUAL AWARENESS: RIGPA

The fundamental reality of mind is pure, non-dual awareness: rigpa. Its essence is one with the essence of all that exists. In practice, it must not be confused with even the subtlest, quietest, and most expansive states of the moving mind. Unrecognized, the nature of mind manifests as the moving mind, but when it is known directly it is both the path to liberation and liberation itself.

Dzogchen teachings often use a mirror to symbolize rigpa. A mirror reflects everything without choice, preference, or judgement. It reflects the beautiful and the ugly, the big and the small, the virtuous and the non-virtuous. There are no limits or restrictions on what it can reflect, yet the mirror is unstained and unaffected by whatever is reflected in it. Nor does it ever cease reflecting.

Similarly, all phenomena of experience arise in rigpa: thoughts, images, emotions, the grasping and the grasped, every apparent subject and object, every experience. The conceptual mind itself arises and abides in rigpa. Life and death take place in the nature of mind, but it is neither born nor does it die, just as reflections come and go without creating or destroying the mirror. Identifying with the conceptual mind, we live as one of the reflections in the mirror, reacting to the other reflections, suffering confusion and pain, endlessly living and dying. We take the reflections for the reality and spend our lives chasing illusions.

When the conceptual mind is free of grasping and aversion, it spontaneously relaxes into unfabricated rigpa. Then there is no longer an identification with the reflections in the mirror and we can effortlessly accommodate all that arises in experience, appreciating every moment. If hatred arises, the mirror is filled with hatred. When love arises, the mirror is filled with love. For the mirror itself, neither love nor hatred is significant: both are equally a manifestation of its innate capacity to reflect. This is known as the mirror-like wisdom; when we recognize the nature of mind and develop the ability to abide in it, no emotional state distracts us. Instead, all states and all phenomena, even anger, jealousy, and so on, are released into the purity and clarity that is their essence. Abiding in rigpa, we cut karma at its root and are released from the bondage of samsara.

Stabilizing in rigpa also makes it easier to realize all other spiritual aspirations. It is easier to practice virtue when free of grasping and the sense of lack, easier to practice compassion when not obsessed with ourselves, easier to practice transformation when unattached to false and constricted identities.

The *Mother Tantra* refers to the nature of mind as "primordial mind." It is like the ocean, while ordinary mind is like the rivers, lakes, and creeks that share in the nature of the ocean and return to it, but temporarily exist as apparently separate bodies of water. The moving mind is also compared to bubbles in the ocean of primordial mind that constantly form and dissolve, depending on the strength of the karmic winds. But the nature of the ocean does not change.

Rigpa arises spontaneously from the base. Its activity is ceaseless manifestation; all phenomena arise in it without disturbing it. The result of abiding wholly in the nature of mind is the three bodies (kayas) of the buddha: the dharmakaya, which is thoughtless essence; the sambhogakaya, which is ceaseless manifestation; and the nirmanakaya, which is undeluded compassionate activity.

Base Rigpa and Path Rigpa

Two types of rigpa are defined in the context of practice. Although only a conceptual division, it is helpful in instruction. The first, the base rigpa, is the pervasive foundational awareness of the base (*khyab-rig*). Every being that has a mind has this awareness—buddhas as well as samsaric beings—as it is from this awareness that all minds arise.

The second is the arising innate awareness of the path (*sam-rig*), which is the individual's experience of the pervasive awareness. It is called path rigpa because it refers to the direct experience of rigpa that yogis have when they enter the practice of Dzogchen and receive the introduction, initiation, and transmission. That is, it is not realized in experience until the practitioner is introduced to it.

The potential for path rigpa to manifest lies in the fact that our minds arise from the primordial awareness of the base. When the primordial awareness is known directly, we call it innate awareness, and this is the path rigpa the yogi knows. In this context, we refer to the primordial pure awareness as rigpa, and the rigpa that arises on the path as *rang-rig*. The first is like cream and the second like butter in the sense that they are of the same substance but something must be done to produce the butter. This is arising or path rigpa because we enter it, then leave it and fall back into the moving mind. It is intermittent in our experience. But rigpa is always present—the primordial base rigpa *is* presence, neither arising nor ceasing—whether we recognize it or not.

3 The Base: Kunzhi

Kunzhi, the base of all existence, of matter as well as the minds of sentient beings, is the inseparable unity of emptiness and clarity. These two are also called *clear* and *light*, the same clear light of sleep yoga. (The kunzhi in the Dzogchen teaching is not synonymous with the kunzhi as it is referred to in the sutric *Cittamatra* school, where kunzhi or *alayavijnana* describes a neutral but unawakened mental consciousness that contains all categories of thought and karmic traces.)

The essence of kunzhi is emptiness (*sunyata*). It is unlimited, absolute space; it is empty of entities, inherent existence, concepts, and boundaries. It is the empty space that seems to be external to us, the empty space that objects inhabit, and the empty space of the mind. Kunzhi has neither inside nor outside, cannot be said to exist (for it is nothing), nor not to exist (for it is reality itself). It is limitless, cannot be destroyed or created, was not born, and does not die. Language used to describe it is necessarily paradoxical, since kunzhi is beyond dualism and concept. Any linguistic construction that attempts to comprehend it is already in error and can only point to that which it cannot encompass.

The clarity or light aspect of kunzhi, on the level of the individual, is rigpa, pure awareness. The kunzhi is sky-like, but it is not the same as the sky, which lacks awareness, because kunzhi is awareness as well as emptiness. This is not to suggest that kunzhi is a subject aware "of," but rather that the awareness is the emptiness. The emptiness is the clarity, the clarity is the emptiness. There is neither subject nor object in kunzhi, nor any other duality or distinction.

When the sun goes down in the evening, we say that darkness falls. This is darkness from the perceiver's point of view. Space is always clear and pervasive, it does not change when the sun rises or sets; there is not dark space and light space. It is only dark or light for us, the perceiver. The darkness takes place in the space but does not affect the space. When the lamp of awareness is lit, the space of kunzhi, the base, is illuminated for us, but the kunzhi was never dark. The darkness was the result of obscurations; our awareness was entangled in the darkness of the ignorant mind.

MIND AND MATTER

The essence of both mind and matter is kunzhi, so why does matter lack awareness? Why can sentient beings become enlightened and matter cannot? In Dzogchen we explain this with a crystal and a lump of coal, where crystal represents mind and coal represents matter.

When the sun shines, the coal, even though drenched in light, cannot radiate that light. It lacks the capacity, just as matter lacks the reflective capacity of innate awareness. But when the sunlight reaches the crystal, it reflects the light because it has the innate capacity to do so; that is its nature. This capacity manifests as displays of multi-hued light. Similarly, sentient beings have the capacity of innate awareness. The mind of a sentient being reflects the light of primordial awareness and its potential is displayed in either the projections of mind or in the pure light of rigpa.

4 Knowing

In sutric Buddhism, it is taught that the ordinary person cannot know emptiness through direct perception, but must rely on inferential cognition. There is a great deal of discussion both historically and currently in sutric traditions regarding how to employ inferential cognition and reason toward the recognition of emptiness, but little about recognition of the nature of mind through the senses. In sutra, only the yogi who has attained the third path, the path of seeing, has yogic direct perception of emptiness, at which time he or she is no longer categorized as an ordinary being.

Dzogchen has a different view. The teachings tell us that not only can the emptiness and clarity of the nature of mind be directly apprehended through the senses, but that it is easier and more valid to use the senses in this spiritual task than to use the conceptual mind. The senses are the immediate gates of direct perception, which, before it is seized by the conceptual mind, is very close to pure awareness. Some sutric commentaries criticize Dzogchen, saying that Dzogchen practitioners are too caught up in visions of light and so on, visions that even ordinary beings can have. But this is as it should be; the nature of mind that we are recognizing exists in all beings.

Often, relying on the intellect for understanding, we become satisfied with concepts. We can be conditioned to assume, upon hearing certain words, that we understand what is meant without ever having had direct experience of what the word indicates. Instead of relying on direct apprehension of the truth behind the concept, we consult the conceptual models we have constructed of that which we wish to understand. This makes it easy to stay lost in the moving mind; it is mistaking the map for the territory, or the finger pointing at the moon for the moon itself. While we may end up with an impressive description of the truth, we also end up not living in that truth.

The nature of the mind can be experienced through the eye sense consciousness, the ear sense consciousness, the nose sense consciousness, and so on. We see through the eye, but our eye is not seeing. We hear through the ear, but the ear is not hearing. In the same way, the nature of the mind can be experienced through the eye sense consciousness, but it is not the eye sense consciousness that is experiencing.

It is similar with all direct perceptions. The form that is received by the eye sense consciousness and the form that the conceptual mind thinks that the eye sense consciousness has perceived are different. The form that is apprehended directly by the eye sense consciousness is closer to fundamental reality than the modeling of that perception, which takes place in the conceptual mind. The conceptual mind is incapable of direct perception; it recognizes things only through projected mental images and through language, which is itself inferential.

For example, eye sense consciousness sees the phenomena that we call "table." What it perceives is not a "table," but a vivid, sensory experience of light and color. The conceptual mind does not directly perceive the raw and vital phenomena that make up the experience of the eye sense consciousness. Instead it creates a mental image of what the eye consciousness experiences. It claims that it is seeing the table but what it sees is a mental image of the table. This is the critical point where conceptual mind and direct perception differ. When the eye is closed, the "table" can no longer be directly perceived, and that set of phenomena is no longer part of the experience of the immediate sensory present, but the conceptual mind can still project an image of the table, which will not be the same as the directly perceived phenomena. The conceptual mind does not need to stay oriented in the sensual present, but can exist in its own fabrications.

This capacity of the conceptual mind to model direct experience, though of inestimable value to us as humans, is the cause of one of the most insistent obstacles in practice. Before and after direct experience of the nature of mind, the conventional mind attempts to conceptualize the experience. Just as the experience of rigpa is, in the beginning, obscured by forms, thoughts, and a dualistic relationship to the phenomena of experience, so the conceptualization of rigpa becomes a barrier. We can then think we know the nature of mind when we are only experiencing a relationship to a concept.

This is not to say that direct sensory experience is itself the nature of mind. Even with very raw perception we tend to be subtly identified with a perceiving subject, and the experience remains dualistic. But in the very first moment of contact between awareness and the object of the senses, the naked nature of mind is there. For instance, when we are sharply surprised, there is a moment when all our senses are open; we have not identified ourselves as the experiencer or the experience. Normally that moment is a kind of unconsciousness, because the gross moving mind with which we identify has, just for that moment, been shocked into stillness. But if we remain in the awareness of that moment, there is neither perceiver nor perceived, only pure perception: no thought, no mental process, no reaction on the part of a subject to the stimulus of an object. There is only open, nondual awareness. That is the nature of the mind. That is rigpa.

5   Recognizing Clarity and Emptiness

The experience of the non-dual awareness of rigpa is quite wonderful. It is freedom from the restless striving of the samsaric mind. It is not a dull peace, but the opposite. It is pure wakefulness. It is light, open, radiant, and blissful. When we are no longer preoccupied with self-centered pursuits based on the insecurities of the illusory self and its desires and aversions, the world arises in the purity of the natural state in a vivid, pristine display of beauty. For the practitioner stable in rigpa, all experiences arise as an ornamentation of the nature of mind, rather than as a problem or delusion.

But recognizing rigpa is not like taking a drug or having some kind of high experience. It is not something found by performing an action or by altering oneself. It is not a trance or a far-out vision or blinding light. It is what we already have, what we already are. When there is expectation about rigpa, it cannot be found. The expectation is about a fantasy; we look past what is already present. What can be expected from emptiness? Nothing. If there is expectation, only frustration will follow.

Experience of emptiness is like experience of space. In the direct recognition of space, the recognition itself is luminosity. That is rigpa. Not knowing this is *ma-rigpa*, ignorance, our samsaric mind. Space is a good analogy to use, because there is nothing to reference in space. It has value though it is nothing: in it can be built a stupa or a house. Anything can be built if there is the space for it. Space is pure potentiality. It has no up or down, in or out, boundaries or limitations. Those are all qualities we conceptualize in space, not qualities of space itself. There is little that we can say about space, so we normally describe it in terms of what it isn't. This is the same as emptiness; though it is the essence of all that exists, nothing can be affirmed about it because it is beyond all qualities, attributes, or references.

There is nothing more than what is present right now, wherever we are, whatever we are doing. Look up: the empty essence is right there. Look left, right, behind, inside: the empty essence is there. Rigpa, the nature of our own mind, knows the essence and is it. Sometimes we feel a strong desire for spiritual experience. That is good: we can generate compassion, do visualization, practice generosity, or do many other practices. We can work with the conceptual side of the path or develop certain qualities in ourselves. But rigpa cannot be worked with. If we do not know the base where we are right now, then we cannot find it until we stop looking for it.

On one level, delusion does not exist and never has. The base of everything is and has always been pure. This direct realization is always accessible, but is unknown to the individual. When we enter the path, we try to obtain this knowledge. But trying has to do with thought and effort, and trying, thought, and effort—in one sense—work against the realization of rigpa. Rigpa is found when no effort is put out, not even the effort to be a self. Rigpa is the complete absence of effort, it is unfabricated and spontaneously perfect. It is the stillness in which activity occurs, the silence in which sound occurs, the thoughtless space in which thought occurs. Having to try is the karmic effect of ignorance—we are paying off the karma of habitual ignorance by trying to understand. But rigpa is outside of karma, it is the awareness of the base, and karma takes place in the base. When we recognize and realize rigpa, we no longer identify with the karmic mind.

What we search for is closer to us than our own thoughts, than our own experience, because clear light is the ground of all experience. So, when we refer to the "experience of clear light," what do we mean? It is not really an experience at all, but rather the space in which subjectivity, sleep, dream, and waking experience occur. We sleep and dream in the luminosity of the kunzhi, the essence of wakefulness, rather than have an experience of kunzhi in us. It is only from our limited perspective that we think of it as an experience that we have.

When the moving mind dissolves into the pure awareness of rigpa, we see the light that has always been, we realize what we already are. We may then think that it is "our experience," that it is something that we made by practicing. But it is the space in which experience arises recognizing itself. This is the son rigpa knowing the mother rigpa, pure awareness knowing itself.

BALANCE

Normally clear light is spoken of in positive terms—emptiness and clarity or openness and luminosity. Although these two aspects are a unity that has never been separated, as an aid to practice we can think of these as two qualities that must be balanced.

Emptiness without awareness is like the sleep of ignorance: a blankness devoid of experience, empty of all discriminations, entities, and so on, but also empty of awareness. Clarity without emptiness is like extreme agitation in which the phenomena of experience are taken to be substantial entities, physical and mental, that impinge on our awareness with the insistence of a fever dream. At night this state results in insomnia. Neither extreme is good. We must balance these so that we neither lose awareness nor are trapped in the illusion that what arises in awareness is solid and independently existing.

DISCRIMINATION

Rigpa is never lost and it is never not rigpa. The very ground of our being is pervasive, self-existing, empty, primordial awareness. But each of us must ask ourselves whether we know this primordial awareness directly or are we distracted from it by the movement of the temporal mind? And each of us must answer for ourselves; no one can tell us the answer.

When we are involved in internal processes, we are not in rigpa, for rigpa has no process. Process is a function of the conceptual moving mind; rigpa is effortless.

Rigpa is like the early morning sky: pure, expansive, spacious, clear, awake, fresh, and quiet. Although rigpa does not actually have any qualities or attributes, these are the qualities against which the teachings suggest the practitioner check his or her experience.

6 Self

The word *self* has been defined differently by various religions and philosophies from ancient times to the present. Bön-Buddhism places a great emphasis on the doctrine of no-self or emptiness (sunyata), which is the ultimate truth of all phenomena. Without understanding emptiness it is difficult to cut the root of the egoic self and to find liberation from its boundaries.

However, when we read about the spiritual journey we also read about self-liberation and self-realization. And we certainly seem to be a self. We can argue to convince others that we do not have a self, but when our life is threatened or something is taken from us, the self that we claim does not exist can become quite afraid or upset.

According to Bön-Buddhism, the conventional self does exist. Otherwise no one would create karma, suffer, and find liberation. It is the inherent self that does not exist. Lack of an inherent self means that there is no core discrete entity that is unchanging through time. Though the nature of mind does not change, it should not be confused with a discrete entity, a "self," a little bit of indestructible awareness that is "me." The nature of mind is not an individual's possession and is not an individual. It is the nature of sentience itself and is the same for all sentient beings.

Let us again refer to the example of reflections in a mirror. If we focus on the reflections, we can say there is this reflection and that other reflection, pointing to two different images. They grow larger and smaller, come and go, and we can follow them around in the mirror as if they were separate beings. They are like the conventional self. However, the reflections are not discrete entities, they are a play of light, unsubstanced illusions in the empty luminosity of the mirror. They exist as separate entities only through conceptualizing them as such. The reflections are a manifestation of the nature of the mirror, just as the conventional self is a manifestation that arises from, abides in, and dissolves back into the empty limpidity of the base of existence, kunzhi.

The conventional self with which you normally identify and the moving mind which gives rise to it are both fluid, dynamic, provisional, substanceless, mutable, impermanent, and lacking in inherent existence, like the reflection in the mirror. You can see this in your own life if you examine it. Imagine filling out forms with information about yourself. You list your name, gender, age, address, job, relationship status, and physical description. You take tests that describe your personality traits and I.Q. You write down your goals and dreams, beliefs, thoughts, values, and fears.

Now imagine all those things taken away. What is left? Take away more—your friends and home, your country and clothes. You lose the ability to speak or to think with language. You lose your memories. You lose your senses. Where is your self? Is it your body? What if you lose your arms and legs, live with a mechanical heart and a lung machine, suffer brain damage and lose mental functions. At what point do you stop being a self? If you keep peeling away layers of identity and hierarchies of attributes, at some point there is nothing left.

You are not the self you were when you were one year old, or ten. You are not the self you were even an hour ago. There is nothing that does not change. At death, the last remnants of what seems to be an unchanging self are gone. When reborn, you may be a different type of being altogether, with a different body, different gender, different mental capacity. It is not that you are not an individual—obviously you are—but that all individuals lack inherent, independent existence. The conventional self is radically contingent, existing as a moment-to-moment fabrication like the stream of thoughts that endlessly arise in the clarity of the mind, or the unceasing manifestations of images in the mirror. Thoughts exist as thoughts, but when they are examined in meditation they dissolve into the emptiness from which they arose. It is the same with the conventional self: when deeply examined, it proves only to be a concept ascribed to a loosely defined collection of constantly changing events. And just as thoughts continue to arise, so do our provisional identities. Erroneously identifying with the conventional self and taking oneself to be a subject surrounded by objects is the foundation of dualistic vision and is the root dichotomy upon which the endless suffering of samsara is founded.

7 Paradox of the Essenceless Self

But how, if the base of the individual is pure, empty awareness, can a conventional self and a moving mind exist at all? Here is an example based on experiences we all have: when we dream, an entire world manifests in which we can have any kind of experience. During the dream we are identified with one subject, but there are other beings, apparently separate from us, having their own experiences and seeming as real as the self we take ourselves to be. There is also an apparent material world: the floors hold us up, our body has sensations, we can eat and touch.

When we wake, we realize that the dream was only a projection of our mind. It took place in our mind and was made of the energy of our mind. But we were lost in it, reacting to the mind-created images as if they were real and outside of ourselves. Our mind is able to create a dream and to identify with one being that it places in the dream, while disidentifying with others. We can even identify with subjects that are far different than we are in our daily life.

As ordinary beings, we are, in the same way, identified right now with a conventional self that is also a projection of mind. We relate to apparent objects and entities that are further mind projections. The base of existence (kunzhi) has the capacity to manifest everything that exists, even beings that become distracted from their true nature, just as our mind can project beings that are apparently separate from us in a dream. When we wake, the dream that is our conventional self dissolves into pure emptiness and luminous clarity.

Final Words

The practices of dream and sleep are not common practices for Tibetans. They are not normally given to young practitioners, nor are they taught to the general public. But things have changed. I am teaching these things because so many people in the West have an interest in dreams and dreaming, and in dream work. Usually this interest is psychological; I hope by presenting these teachings that dream work might progress to something deeper. Psychological dream work may create more happiness in samsara and that is good, but if full realization is the goal then something more must be done. This is where sleep yoga is particularly important. It is fully at the heart of the practice of the Great Perfection, Dzogchen, which could be summarized thus: every moment of life—waking, dreaming, and sleeping—abide in pure non-dual awareness. This is the certain road to enlightenment and the path that all realized masters have taken. This is the essence of sleep yoga.

How can you have the experience of clear light? I think it is important to reflect on this question as it has to do with your attitude toward the teaching. All the teachings are of a single essence. I am referring to rigpa, to the clear light. No matter how much you learn, how many texts you study, how many teachings you receive, you will not have gotten the main point if you do not know this single essence. Tibetans have a saying: "You can receive so many teachings that your head is flat from being touched with the initiation vase, but if you don't know the essence, nothing will change."

When one does not directly know the nature of mind, the teachings can be difficult to understand. They may seem to refer to something impossible, because the nature of mind is beyond the conceptual mind and cannot be comprehended by it. Trying to grasp the nature of mind through concepts is like trying to understand the nature of the sun by studying shadows: something can be learned, but the essence remains unknown. This is why practice is necessary, to go beyond the moving mind and to know the nature of mind directly.

Some people come to feel burdened by all the teachings they have accumulated. This is based on a misunderstanding of the path. Continue learning and receiving teachings, but develop a deep enough understanding that you can take from them what supports you. The teachings are not an obligation once you understand and apply them. They are a path to freedom and there is joy in following that path. They only feel like a burden if one becomes mired in their form without understanding their purpose. It is necessary to learn how to conclude the teachings; this is done not through words or concepts, but in experience.

On the other hand, do not allow yourself to become trapped by the practice. What does this mean? If you continue to practice without results, with no positive changes in life, the practice is not working. Do not think that you are doing the practice if you are simply going through the motions without understanding. Empty rituals accomplish little. You need to penetrate the practice with understanding, determine what the essence is and how to apply it.

The dharma really is flexible. But this does not mean that you should throw out the tradition and make up your own. These practices are powerful and effective. They have been the vehicle for countless people to realize liberation. If the practice is not working, experimentation should be done to try to find what the purpose of the practice is. Consulting with your teacher is best. When you understand the practices, you will also find that the form is not the problem; it is the application of the form that needs to be perfected. The practice is here for you, not you for it. Learn the form, understand the purpose of it, apply it in practice, and realize the result.

Where do you ultimately conclude the practice? In the process of death, the intermediate state, the bardo. The bardo after death is like a major airport that everyone has to pass through on their travels. It is the borderline between samsara and nirvana. The capacity to abide in non-dual presence is the passport that allows entry to nirvana. If you have never had the experience of clear light during sleep, it is difficult to pass from samsara in the bardo; it is as if thick sleep covers the clear light, a blanket of thick thought covering rigpa. If you can integrate with the clear light of sleep, then you can integrate with the clear light of death. Integrating with the clear light of sleep is like passing midterm exams; you are doing well and will probably pass the final that is given in the bardo. Integrating with the clear light of death means finding buddha within yourself and being able to realize, directly, that what arises is essenceless appearance.

The presence of rigpa continues from this world into the next, so practice to experience it now, to become it and abide in it. That is the path, the continuity of clarity and unceasing wisdom. All the beings who achieved enlightenment and became buddhas crossed the border and entered the clear light. Know this so that you know what it is you prepare for. Try to get the sense of the whole of the teachings, where you are, and where you are going. Then you will know how to apply them, when to use what, and what the results will be. The teachings are like a map that can tell you where to go, where to find what you are looking for. The map clarifies everything. Without it you can become lost.

Pray to connect with the clear light during death. Pray that everyone connects with the nature of mind at the time of their death. The power of prayer is very great. When you pray, intention is developed, and what you pray for moves toward realization.

Every individual experiences moments of peace and joy. If the clear light seems a distant goal, just try continuously to maintain the positive experiences of peace and joy. Perhaps when you remember the master or the dakini you feel joy, or when you attend to the beauty of the natural world, happiness arises. Make doing these things a practice. Generate gratitude and appreciation during every moment. The clear light is the pinnacle of mystical experience, the highest joy and the greatest peace. So take joy and peace as qualities to maintain, as supports in developing the continuity of awareness. Feel these qualities in the body, see them in the world, and wish them for others. Through doing this you can develop awareness while generating compassion and positive traits.

Continuity is the key to integrating life and practice. With awareness and intention, continuity can be developed. When it is, your life will be different, and you will become a positive influence on the life around you.

Dream and sleep yogas are methods to recognize the clear light and abide in it through all the moments of life: waking, meditating, dreaming, sleeping, and death. Essentially, the teachings are designed to help us to recognize the nature of mind, to understand and overcome the obstacles in our practice, and to abide fully in rigpa. We can utilize the same methods to remain in joy, to find peace in the midst of the turmoil of the world, to live well, and to appreciate each vivid moment of our human existence.

Great masters have written that it has taken them many years of steady practice to accomplish sleep yoga, so do not be discouraged if you have no experience the first or the hundredth time you try it. There are benefits just from attempting the practice. Anything that brings more awareness into your life is beneficial. It takes long, sustained intention and practice to realize the goal. Do not allow yourself to grow discouraged. Bring your entire being to the practice; with strong intention and joyful effort you will surely find your life changing in positive ways and will certainly accomplish the practices.

I hope that those who have read this book will discover a new knowledge of dream and sleep, one that will help improve their daily life and that will ultimately lead to enlightenment.

Appendix: Outline of Dream Yoga Practices

THE FOUR FOUNDATIONAL PRACTICES

Changing the Karmic Traces

Throughout the day, continuously remain in the awareness that all experience is a dream. Encounter all things as objects in a dream, all events as events in a dream, all people as people in a dream. Envision your own body as a transparent illusory body. Imagine you are in a lucid dream during the entire day. Do not allow these reminders to be merely empty repetition. Each time you tell yourself, "This is a dream," actually become more lucid. Involve your body and your senses in becoming more present.

Removing Grasping and Aversion

Encounter all things that create desire and attachment as the illusory, empty, luminous phenomena of a dream. Recognize your reactions to phenomena as a dream; all emotions, judgements, and preferences are being dreamt up. You can be certain that you are doing this correctly if immediately upon remembering that your reaction is a dream, desire and attachment lessen.

Strengthening Intention
Before going to sleep, review the day and reflect on how the practice has been. Let memories of the day arise and recognize them as memories of dream. Develop a strong intention to be aware in the coming night's dreams. Put your whole heart into this intention and pray strongly for success.

Cultivating Memory and Joyful Effort
Begin the day with the strong intention to maintain the practice. Review the night, developing happiness if you remembered or were lucid in your dreams. Recommit yourself to the practice, with the intention to become lucid if you were not, and to further develop lucidity if you were. At any time during the day or evening it is good to pray for success in practice. Generate as strong an intention as possible. This is the key to the practice.

PREPARATORY PRACTICES BEFORE SLEEP
Nine Purifications Breathing
Sitting in meditation posture before lying down to sleep, do the nine purification breaths.

Guru Yoga
Practice guru yoga. Generate strong devotion, then merge your mind with the pure awareness of the master, the ultimate master that is the primordial awareness, your true nature.

Protection
Lie down in the correct posture, men on the right side, women on the left side. Visualize dakinis surrounding you, protecting you. Use imagination to transform the room into a protected, sacred environment. Gentle your breathing and calm your mind, observing it until you are relaxed and present, not caught up in stories and fantasies. Create a strong intention to have vivid, clear dreams, to remember dreams, and to recognize the dream as a dream while you are in it.

THE MAIN PRACTICES
Bringing Awareness into the Central Channels
The practice of the first watch of the night. Focus on the throat center, on the pure, translucent, crystalline *A* that is tinged red from the color of the four red petals upon which it rests. Merge with the red light.

Increasing Clarity

Approximately two hours later, wake. In the same lion posture, practice the breathing seven times. Focus on the white tiglé in the brow chakra as you fall asleep. Allow the white light to dissolve everything, until you and the light are one.

Strengthening Presence

After approximately two more hours, again awaken. Lay back against a high pillow with your legs lightly and comfortably crossed. Focus on the black *HUNG* in the heart chakra. Breathe deeply, fully, and gently twenty-one times. Merge with the black *HUNG* and fall asleep.

Developing Fearlessness

Another two hours later, wake again. No particular posture or breathing is necessary. Focus on a black, luminous tiglé in the secret chakra, behind the genitals. Fall asleep while merged with the black light.

Upon each awakening try to be present and to be with the practice. In the morning, the final waking of the night, immediately be present. Review the night, generate intentions, and continue with the practice during the day.

In addition, it is helpful to make time to do the calm abiding (zhiné) practice during the day. This will help to make the mind quiet and focused and will benefit all other practices.

The most important point of both the preparation and the main practice is to maintain presence as consistently as possible throughout the day and the night. This is the essence of both dream and sleep yogas.

Glossary

bardo (Tib., *bar do;* Skt., *antarabhāva*). Bardo means "in-between state," and refers to any transitional state of existence—life, meditation, dream, death—but most commonly refers to the intermediate state between death and rebirth.

Bön (Tib., *bon*). Bön is the indigenous spiritual tradition of Tibet that predates Indian Buddhism. Although scholars disagree about the origin of Bön, the tradition itself claims an unbroken lineage seventeen thousand years old. Similar to Tibetan Buddhist sects, particularly the Nyingma, Bön is distinguished by a distinctive iconography, a rich shamanistic tradition, and a separate lineage reaching back to the Buddha Shenrab Miwoche rather than to Shakyamuni Buddha.

The nine vehicles of Bön contain teachings on practical matters, such as grammar, astrology, medicine, prognostication, the pacification of spirits and so on, as well as teachings on logic, epistemology, metaphysics, the different levels of tantra, and complete lineages of the Great Perfection (Dzogchen).

chakra (Tib., *khor-lo;* Skt., *cakra*). Literally "wheel" or "circle." Chakra is a Sanskrit word referring to energetic centers in the body. A chakra is a location at which a number of energetic channels (*tsa*) meet. Different meditation systems work with different chakras.

channel (Tib., *tsa;* Skt., *nāḍi*). The channels are the "veins" in the system of energetic circulation in the body, through which stream the currents of subtle energy that sustain and vivify life. The channels themselves are energetic and cannot be found in the physical dimension. However, through practice or natural sensitivity, individuals can become experientially aware of the channels.

chöd (Tib., *gcod*). Literally: "to cut off," or "to cut through." Also known as the "expedient use of fear," and the "cultivation of generosity," chöd is a ritual practice meant to remove all attachment to one's own body and ego by compassionately offering all that one is to other beings. To this end, the practice involves an elaborate evocation of various classes of beings and the subsequent imaginary cutting up and transformation of the practitioner's own body into objects and substances of offering. Chöd uses melodious singing, drums, bells, and horns, and is generally practiced in locations that incite fear, such as charnel grounds, cemeteries, and remote mountain passes.

dakini (Tib., *mkha' gro ma*). The Tibetan equivalent of dakini is *khadroma*, which literally means female sky-traveler. "Sky" refers to emptiness, and the dakini travels in that emptiness; that is, she acts in full realization of emptiness, absolute reality. A dakini can be a human woman who has realized her true nature, or a non-human female or goddess, or a direct manifestation of enlightened mind. Dakini also refers to a class of beings born in the pure realm of the dakinis.

dharma (Tib., *chos*). A very broad term, dharma has many meanings. In the context of this book, dharma is both the spiritual teachings that ultimately derive from the Buddhas and the spiritual path itself. Dharma also means existence.

dharmakaya (Tib., *chos sku*). A buddha is said to possess three bodies (*kaya*): dharmakaya, *sambhogakaya*, and *nirmanakaya*. The dharmakaya, often translated as the "truth body," refers to the absolute nature of the buddha, which all buddhas share in common and which is identical with the absolute nature of all that exists: emptiness. The dharmakaya is non-dual, empty of conceptuality, and free of all characteristics. (See also **sambhogakaya** and **nirmanakaya**.)

Dzogchen (Tib., *rdzogs chen*). The "great perfection" or "great completion." Dzogchen is considered the highest teaching and practice in both Bön and in the Nyingma school of Tibetan Buddhism. Its fundamental tenet is that reality, including the individual, is already complete and perfect, that nothing needs to be transformed (as in *tantra*) or renounced (as in *sutra*) but only recognized for what it truly is. The essential Dzogchen practice is "self-liberation": allowing all that arises in experience to exist just as it is, without elaboration by the conceptual mind, without grasping or aversion.

gong-ter (Tib., *gong gter*). In Tibetan culture there is a tradition of *terma*: sacred objects, texts, or teachings hidden by the masters of one age for the benefit of the future age in which the termas are found. The tantric masters who discover terma are known as *tertons*, treasure finders. Terma have been and may be found in physical locations, such as caves or cemeteries; in elements such as water, wood, earth, or space; or received in dreams, visionary experience, and found directly in deep levels of consciousness. The latter case is known as gong-ter: mind treasure.

guardians (Tib., *srung ma/ chos skyong*; Skt., *dharmapāla*). Guardians are male or female beings pledged to protect the dharma (teachings) and the practitioners of the teachings. They may be worldly protectors or wrathful manifestations of enlightened beings. Tantric practitioners generally propitiate and rely upon guardians associated with their lineage.

jalus (Tib., *'ja lus*). The "rainbow body." The sign of full realization in Dzogchen is the attainment of the rainbow body. The realized Dzogchen practitioner, no longer deluded by apparent substantiality or dualisms such as mind and matter, releases the energy of the elements that compose the physical body at the time of death. The body itself is dissolved, leaving only hair and nails, and the practitioner consciously enters death.

karma (Tib., *las*). Karma means literally "action," but more broadly refers to the law of cause and effect. Any action taken physically, verbally, or mentally, serves as a "seed" that will bear the "fruit" of its consequences in the future when the conditions are right for its realization. Positive actions have positive effects, such as happiness; negative actions have negative effects, such as unhappiness. Karma does not mean that life is determined, but that conditions arise out of past actions.

karmic trace (Tib., *bag chags*). Every action—physical, verbal, or mental—undertaken by an individual, if performed with intention and even the slightest aversion or desire, leaves a trace in the mindstream of that individual. The accumulation of these karmic traces serves to condition every moment of experience of that individual, positively and negatively.

kunzhi (Tib., *kun gzhi*). In Bön, the kunzhi is the base of all that exists, including the individual. It is not synonymous with the *alaya vijnana* of Yogacara, which is more akin to the **kunzhi namshe** (see below). The kunzhi is the unity of emptiness and clarity, of the absolute open indeterminacy of ultimate reality and the unceasing display of appearance and awareness. The kunzhi is the base or ground of being.

kunzhi namshe (Tib., *kun gzhi rnam shes*; Skt., *ālaya vijñāna*). The kunzhi namshe is the basic consciousness of the individual. It is the "repository" or "storehouse" in which the karmic traces are stored, from which future, conditioned experience arises.

lama (Tib., *bla ma*; Skt., *guru*). Lama literally means "highest mother." *Lama* refers to a spiritual teacher, who is of unsurpassed importance to the student practitioner. In the Tibetan tradition, the lama is considered to be more important even than the buddha, for it is the lama that brings the teachings to life for the student. On an ultimate level, the lama is one's own buddha-nature. On the relative level, the lama is one's personal teacher.

loka (Tib., *'jig rten*). Literally "world" or "world system." Commonly used in English to refer to the six realms of cyclic existence, loka actually refers to the greater world systems, one of which is occupied by the six realms. (See **six realms of cyclic existence**.)

lung (Tib., *rlung*, Skt., *vāyu*). Lung is the vital wind energy, commonly known in the West by one of its Sanskrit names, *prana*. Lung has a broad range of meanings; in the context of this book it refers to the vital energy upon which both the vitality of the body and consciousness depend.

ma-rigpa (Tib., *ma rig pa*; Skt., *avidyā*). Ignorance. The lack of knowledge of the truth, of the base, the kunzhi. Often two categories of Ma-rigpa are described: innate ignorance and cultural ignorance.

nirmanakaya (Tib., *sprul sku*; Skt., *nirmāṇakāya*). The nirmanakaya is the "emanation body" of the dharmakaya. Usually this refers to the visible, physical manifestation of a buddha. The term is also resonant with the dimension of physicality.

prana (See **lung**.)

rigpa (Tib., *rig pa*; Skt., *vidyā*). Literally, "awareness" or "knowing." In the Dzogchen teachings, rigpa means awareness of the truth, innate awareness, the true nature of the individual.

rinpoche (Tib., *rin po che*). Literally, "precious one." An honorific widely used in addressing an incarnate lama.

samaya (Tib., *dam tshig*; Skt., *samaya*). Commitment or vow. Commonly, the commitment the practitioner makes in connection with tantric practice, regarding behaviors and actions. There are general vows and vows specific to particular tantric practices.

sambhogakaya (Tib., *longs sku*; Skt., *sambhogakāya*). The "enjoyment body" of the buddha. The sambhogakaya is a body made entirely of light. This form is often visualized in tantric and sutric practices. In Dzogchen, more often the image of the dharmakaya is visualized.

samsara (Tib., *'khor ba*). The realm of suffering that arises from the occluded, dualistic mind, where all entities are impermanent, lack inherent existence, and where all sentient beings are subject to suffering. Samsara includes the six realms of cyclic existence, but more broadly refers to the characteristic mode of existence of sentient beings who suffer through being trapped in the delusions of ignorance and duality. Samsara ends when a being attains full liberation from ignorance, nirvana.

Shenla Odker (Tib., *gShen lHa 'od dkar*). Shenla Odker is the sambhogakaya form of Shenrab Miwoche, the buddha who founded Bön.

Shenrab Miwoche (Tib., *gShen rab mi bo che*). Shenrab Miwoche was the nirmanakaya Buddha that founded Bön, traditionally believed to have lived seventeen thousand years ago. There are fifteen volumes of biography of Shenrab Miwoche in the Bön literature.

six realms of cyclic existence (Tib., *rigs drug*). Commonly referred to as "the six realms" or "six lokas." The six realms refer to six classes of beings: gods, demi-gods, humans, animals, hungry-ghosts, and hell-beings. Beings in the six realms are subject to suffering. They are literal realms, in which beings take birth, and also broad experiential and affective bands of potential experience that shape and limit experience even in our current life.

sutra (Tib., *mdo*). The sutras are texts composed of teachings that came directly from the historical Buddha. The teachings of sutra are based on the path of renunciation and form the base of monastic life.

tantra (Tib., *rgyud*). Tantras are teachings of the Buddhas, as are sutras, but many tantras were rediscovered by yogis of the terma tradition. Tantras are based on the path of transformation and include practices such as working with the energy of the body, the transference of consciousness, dream and sleep yogas, and so on. Certain classes of tantras, of the non-gradual transformation path, may also contain teachings on Dzogchen.

Tapihritsa (Tib., *ta pi hri tsa*). Although considered a historical person, Tapihritsa is iconographically represented as a dharmakaya Buddha, naked and without ornaments, personifying absolute reality. He is one of the two principle masters in the Dzogchen lineage of the Zhang Zhung Nyan Gyud.

three root poisons. These are ignorance, aversion, and desire, the three fundamental afflictions that perpetuate the continuity of life in the realms of suffering.

tiglé (Tib., *thig le*; Skt., *bindu*). Tiglé has multiple meanings depending on context. Although usually translated as "drop" or "seminal point," in the context of dream and sleep yogas the tiglé refers to a luminous sphere of light representing a quality of consciousness and used as a focus in meditation practice.

tsa (See **channel.**)

yidam (Tib., *yid dam*; Skt., *devatā*). The yidam is a tutelary or meditational deity embodying an aspect of enlightened mind. There are four categories yidams: peaceful, increasing, powerful, and wrathful. Yidams manifest in these different forms to overcome specific negative forces.

yogi (Tib., *rnal 'byor pa*). A male practitioner of meditative yogas, such as the dream and sleep yogas.

yogini (Tib., *rnal 'byor ma*). A female practitioner of meditative yoga.

Zhang Zhung Nyan Gyud (Tib., *Zhang Zhung snyan rgyud*). The Zhang Zhung Nyan Gyud is one of the most important cycles of Dzogchen teachings in Bön. It belongs to the *upadesha* series of teachings.

zhiné (Tib., *zhi gnas*; Skt., *śamatha*). "Calm abiding" or "tranquility." The practice of calm abiding uses focus on an external or internal object to develop concentration and mental stability. Calm abiding is a fundamental practice, the basis for the development of all other higher meditation practices, and is necessary for both dream and sleep yogas.

Bibliography

TIBETAN TEXTS

Ma rgyud Sangs rgyas rgyud gsum
  1: *Ma rgyud thugs rje nyi ma'i gnyid pa lam du khyer ba'i 'grel pa*
  2: *Ma rgyud thug rje nyi ma'i rmi ba lam du khyer ba'i Hgrel pa*

A-khrid thun-mtshams bcu-lnga dang cha-lag bcas

Zhang Zhung Nyan rgyud bka' rgyud skor bzhi

BOOKS IN ENGLISH

Dalai Lama. *Sleeping, Dreaming, and Dying: An Exploration of Consciousness with the Dalai Lama.* Edited and narrated by Francisco Varela. Translations by B. Alan Wallace and Thupten Jinpa. Boston: Wisdom Publications, 1997.

Shardza Tashi Gyaltsen. *Heart Drops of Dharmakaya: Dzogchen Practice of the Bön Tradition.* Translation and commentary by Lopon Tenzin Namdak. Ithaca: Snow Lion Publications, 1993.

Namkhai Norbu Rinpoche. *Dream Yoga and the Practice of Natural Light.* Edited and introduced by Michael Katz. Ithaca: Snow Lion Publications, 1992.

Venerable Gyatrul Rinpoche. *Ancient Wisdom: Nyingma Teachings on Dream Yoga, Meditation, and Transformation.* Root text translations by B. Alan Wallace. Commentary translations by Sangye Khandro. Ithaca: Snow Lion Publications, 1993.

ALSO BY TENZIN WANGYAL RINPOCHE

Tenzin Wangyal Rinpoche. *The Wonders of the Natural Mind.* Foreword by H. H. the Dalai Lama. Barrytown: Station Hill Press, 1993.

Tenzin Wangyal Rinpoche teaches at several locations in the United States, Mexico, and Europe. If you would like information on his and other teachers' schedules, please contact:

The Ligmincha Institute
P. O. Box 1892
Charlottesville, Virginia 22903 USA

Phone: (804) 977-6161
Fax: (804) 977-7020
Web Page: http://www.comet.net/ligmincha/
E-mail: ligmincha@aol.com